Atkins Diet Mistakes You Wish You Knew

Mirsad Hasic

Copyright © Mirsad Hasic

All rights reserved.

ISBN: 1492734373
ISBN-13: 978-1492734376

DEDICATION

I dedicate this book to my wife.

CONTENTS

	Acknowledgments	i
1	This is a True Lifestyle, Not Just a Diet	1
2	Preparing for Atkins	Pg 4
3	Induction	Pg 7
4	Fighting The Induction Flu	Pg 10
5	The Faulty Science of Calories in, Calories out	Pg 13
6	The Scale isn't Your Concern	Pg 16
7	High Fat Intake and Why Fat is Glorious	Pg 19
8	The Phases of Atkins Are Incredibly Important	Pg 22
9	Induction, Reloaded	Pg 25
10	Phase Two, Ongoing Weight Loss	Pg 28
11	Phase Three, Pre-Maintenance	Pg 31
12	Phase Four is More Intense	Pg 34
13	Food Intolerances	Pg 37
14	High Protein Intake and The Atkins Approach	Pg 39
15	Kidney Problems and The Atkins Approach	Pg 41
16	Sweeteners	Pg 44

17	Packaged Shakes, Bars, and Meals	Pg 46
18	Apetite Control	Pg 48
19	Dining Out	Pg 51
20	Sugar Cravings	Pg 54
21	Healthy Fats	Pg 57
22	Thyroid Problems	Pg 60
23	Don't Ignore The Power of Potassium	Pg 63
24	Don't Skip The Magnesium	Pg 66
25	Vitamin D	Pg 68
26	Calcium	Pg 71
27	Iron and The Atkins Diet	Pg 73
28	Sodium Intake	Pg 75
29	Fiber and The Atkins Diet	Pg 78
30	Caffeine	Pg 80
31	Alcohol on Atkins -- Worth Looking Into	Pg 83
32	The Fat Fast	Pg 85
33	Gallbladder Issues	Pg 88
34	Sleep Issues	Pg 90
35	Men's Health	Pg 93

36	Women's Health	Pg 95
37	Pregnancy	Pg 97
38	Depression Issues	Pg 99
39	Net Carbs	Pg 101
40	Actions Stesp for Your New Atkins Life	Pg 103

ACKNOWLEDGMENTS

I would like to thank my family for their support.

1 THIS IS A TRUE LIFESTYLE, NOT JUST A DIET

I am a lot of things: passionate researcher, science geek, and a friend to any and all who are struggling to lose weight and get healthy.

Maybe you are someone who has a lot of weight to lose, and if so, I can completely understand where you're coming from on that.

Or perhaps you only have a few stubborn pounds to shed, and if so, I can understand where you're coming from on that too.

I've had both situations to deal with in my life, and I've found that each one has its own problems.

As much as you might be looking for a quick solution, there really isn't one.

There are so many different answers being bandied about for the same question, that being: just how do we handle obesity as a global society?

I don't profess to have all of the answers, and the science is definitely divided on the subject as well. According to the National Center for Health Statistics

(NCHS), the number of adults who are technically obese has literally doubled over the last 30 years.

That was from a report published back in 2004. (1)

The Atkins Diet is formally known as the Atkins Nutritional Approach, created by Dr. Robert Atkins in 1974.

The focus is completely on carbohydrate-restriction at its foundation, but the diet actually covers so more than just watching your carb intake.

In fact, I discovered such a lot about the Atkins diet through research - and my later adventures by actually embracing the diet t - hat I wanted to share all of my insights with you.

I cover a mix of peer-reviewed journals, traditional news outlets, and premium subject blogs, so as to give you a perspective like no other. (2)

So read on, dear reader, read on.

If you're looking to achieve weight loss success and avoid those mistakes that so many before you have made when attempting the Atkins Diet, then this book is definitely the right choice.

Furthermore, if you're just someone who is simply trying to get healthier, this book is still the right one for you.

Why?

Well, I talk about the real issues that Atkins followers, and low carb followers in general, really need to know about.

There is nothing as rewarding and motivational as being able to claim the health benefits that you deserved from the outset.

Atkins may seem complicated at first, but I'm here to take the mystery out of it.

I don't want anyone left feeling like they can't do this diet and successfully turn it into a way of life.

That's really the end goal with all of my books on diet, fitness, and healthy living.

I want you to see my approach as stepping stones that lead to a healthier and happier lifestyle, rather than just something which is temporary, as is the case with so many other approaches towards diet.

Most weight loss plans, when followed correctly, usually result in some short-term weight loss, but I'd rather you learn how to keep the weight off and successfully maintain the 'new you' for life.

Next up: Preparing for your new Atkins-flavored life, of course!

2 PREPARING FOR ATKINS

Getting ready for the Atkins lifestyle means you will need to clear out your kitchen, get all of your new foods ready, and prepare for a new routine.

Of course, this can be said for just about any diet.

However, I would argue that when it comes to making Atkins work with real effectiveness, the key here is to prepare well.

I have found from my own personal experience that whenever I don't plan out my low-carb meals, I fall into the trap of automatically reaching for higher carb fare.

Needless to say that this does nothing to help me achieve my goals and it wouldn't help you either.

This is why planning is so critical to your success when adopting the Atkins way of life. (3)

So, what do I mean exactly when I say clearing out your kitchen?

Well, you will need to look at the acceptable foods as outlined by Atkins, and then get rid all those items that are not 'Atkins friendly'.

Generally speaking, high-carb items like bread, pasta, sugary yogurt, conventional soda, potatoes, bananas, and more besides, need to be removed.

Such foods are far too high in carbohydrates, and they have no role to play in your new eating plan.

There are some low carb products specifically designed to keep you moving forward on Atkins, but you can look at those at a later time.

For now, you need to keep planning as simple as possible.

One thing that people tend to overlook about Atkins is that they're really moving up (or down) a carbohydrate ladder.

Although it's a low-carb diet, you're not on so few carbs that you will never again have a fulfilling meal on your own terms.

It just means that you're going to become a lot more mindful about what you do eat.

The first phase of Atkins is known as "Induction", which is designed to give you a definite boost in terms of weight loss.

There is quite a lengthy list of foods that can be eaten on Induction, and will truly feel like you've been spoilt for choice.

You will find buttery shrimps all the way up to juicy crab legs and even bacon!

Given the green light to indulge in these once forbidden foods, who wouldn't feel excited about starting on a new diet? (4), (5)

Fill your fridge with plenty of meat, eggs, dairy (including cheese), butter, leafy greens, seafood, and good cooking oils.

Sugar though, should be off your list when getting into Atkins.

It is very high in terms of carbohydrates, and consuming it simply makes you crave for more of the same.

So, in order to succeed with the Atkins diet, it's important to realize that sugar is not your friend in any way, shape, or form.

Just know that sugar is not going to help you lose weight, and it's certainly not going to help you improve your health.

Don't worry; I'm not sentencing you to a lifetime of non-sweet food.

You just have to tweak the way you eat, that's all. (6)

Up next: I'll be talking about that very important early phase of Atkins - The Induction.

3 INDUCTION

If there is one phase of the Atkins Nutritional Approach that will get you moving forward on the path towards weight loss for life, it would be Induction.

However, a lot of people - including Atkins, Inc. themselves - say that this is an optional phase.

If you don't want to do it, however, you don't have to. Dr. Atkins was a firm believer in the Induction phase (as outlined in the Dr. Atkins New Diet Revolution book, and again in the Atkins 72 publication).

He considered it an important phase for anyone who was preparing to follow this way of eating. (7)

My own thoughts are simple; if you really want to feel all the benefits of Atkins, then you need to do the Induction phase.

It's not just something that sounds good, but something you need to do.

There are many reasons why I say this, but most importantly, it's your health that's on the line if you skip this vital phase.

Whenever we can see quick progress, it's like getting a pat on the back, an indication that what we're doing is actually working.

I'm not immune to the way diets do or don't work.

I have plenty of friends that have tried diet after diet and felt like there was just no hope.

I have always suggested Atkins Induction to them because it's a healthy way of losing weight. (8)

The key behind the Induction Phase of Atkins is simple: ketosis.

This is NOT ketoacidosis as some circles suggest.

That is a dangerous condition for Type 1 diabetics where the body produces an extremely high level of ketones that cannot be used as energy.

Ketoacidosis is completely different from ketosis, otherwise known as benign dietary ketosis.

Ketosis is a mild release of ketone bodies rather than a major flood of them into the bloodstream and urine. (9)

If you are non-diabetic, then you're making sufficient insulin so the chances of ketoacidosis are, in all honesty, extremely low.

Ketosis supporters say they experience an extreme burst of energy which helps them get through their day to day tasks without having to reach for coffee or other stimulants just to keep them going.

This feeling of increased energy is exactly what led me to give Atkins a try. I was definitely not disappointed.

To make the Induction phase work, you're going to need to keep your carb intake to 20 grams or less per day.

In fact, you will need to derive most of your carbs through veggies.

It is possible to get your carbohydrates from other sources, but this really isn't a good idea.

It is much better to get your carbs from vegetables due to the high amount of fiber found in most types of edible plants.

This will help to keep you regular as you adapt into your new life on Atkins.

You will also want to stick with it for at least two weeks.

Should you find that Induction is working well for you, and you have quite a bit of weigh to lose, then there's nothing wrong with staying on this phase for a much longer period of time.

Is it going to be restrictive?

In some ways, yes: you will need to avoid most sources of carbohydrates and keep your portions reasonably small.

But to me, this is the "core" of Atkins as we are reshaping the way we see the role food plays within our everyday lives.

There's still plenty of great food that falls in line with Induction, meaning you can go out there and experience a whole new range of flavors!

Up next: I will be talking about the Induction flu, and how to avoid it; a classic problem that faces many Atkins followers.

4 FIGHTING THE INDUCTION FLU

Low-carbing is a great way to lose weight and regain health, but that doesn't mean there aren't any bumps in the road along the way.

A lot of people see weight loss as something linear, but it's really anything but.

You just need to make sure that you're looking at the bigger picture here, and not just see what you want to see.

You might believe, for example, that you can't get the "Induction flu", only to find later that it hits you head on.

For those that don't know what I'm talking about, the Induction flu is something that usually strikes within the first few weeks of committing to a totally low carb way of living.

The adjustment period occurs because the body is moving into ketosis; a process where the body burns fat for energy rather than glucose. (10)

The Induction flu is experienced by marked periods of brain fog, low energy levels, and digestive issues.

How bad it gets all depends on where your carb intake was before you came into Atkins.

If you were someone that hit the fast food places three times a day, then going into the Induction phase will likely be a sharper adjustment than you might have expected.

Be sure to take in plenty of water during this time.

The body will not starve without you eating glucose as it can make this all important energy source from proteins and fats. It's a process called gluconeogenesis.

It's pretty neat to realize that we don't need to consume glucose as our bodies are more than capable of creating it.

This means that the days of having to deal with starchy carbs - that did nothing for you anyway - are fast coming to an end. (12)

If you're dealing with the induction flu right now, keep reading as there are some things you can do that will help you to get through it.

In the very beginning of a low carb diet, fat quickly becomes your friend.

It's a great way to feel full, as well as being a wonderful way to transport much needed nutrients into your cells.

There are fat soluble vitamins that your body needs, and fat and cholesterol go together - in a healthy way - to help regulate your hormones. (13)

If you don't feel up to exercising, or simply don't have the energy to push yourself on workout days, then slow down.

A gentle walk through the park is much kinder on the body than going for a full-fledged run when you barely have the energy to stand up straight.

Remember that Atkins encourages the consumption of butter, which has butyric acid in it, as well as arachidonic acid.

Both of these fatty acids team up to actually improve your mood as well as boost your energy at the same time.

You will soon start to feel like a new person.

The adaptation period, however, varies between individuals.

Some people will go two or three weeks before they're actually capable of being in the "zone" of a true fat burner. (11)

When I was just starting out, I have to admit the "low carb flu" really hit me hard.

Luckily in Sweden, we have access to some pretty good butter, which I relied heavily in order to keep my fat intake high.

Worried about calories?

Don't be.

In the next chapter I will be discussing exactly why "calories in, calories out" doesn't matter when it comes to living life the Atkins way.

5 THE FAULTY SCIENCE OF CALORIES IN, CALORIES OUT

If I had a silver coin for every time I've been told to just eat less and move more, I would have a whole shed full of loose change by now.

This is because the science behind calories in, and calories out (CICO), just doesn't work in the way we've been told it does.

You see, the entire concept of CICO is derived from an old study that just isn't relevant anymore.

It is an attempt to apply the Laws of Thermodynamics to human beings.

This simply doesn't work in practice because humans aren't really a closed system.

There is no way to truly measure all of the variables that would even make CICO valid.

For example, is there a consistent factor that says how an apple is burned in the body?

The answer is no, not really.

The food we consume is going to be burned differently depending on the metabolism of the person eating it.

You cannot just pool humans together under such a theory because it just doesn't hold water when you really look at it logically.

The history of calculating calories is simple: burning the food in a bomb calorimeter (a thick-walled steel container) and then measuring how much heat it produces.

Within our bodies there is no furnace doing that.

We consume energy but we don't necessarily produce it under the origin of the calorie theory.

The food we consume needs to be used by a wide variety of systems, including bacteria found in the gut, and there's no way to really measure how much is consumed by the bacteria.

When you start looking at this from a scientific point of view, it becomes obvious that what we view as a calorie doesn't quite exist. (14)

When we look at this through the lens of the Atkins diet, the reality is that you're going to be taking in a lot of food.

But by restricting your carbs, you're avoiding the weight gain due to insulin dysregulation.

The truth is that the more carbs we take in, the more glucose (sugar) invades the body.

If insulin levels stay constantly elevated, then fat storage is the conclusion.

The insulin hypothesis is gaining momentum, to the point where we now have a way of helping those people who have been overweight for years, actually lose the excess and keep it off for the first time in their lives.

So just how does this connect back to you, the newcomer to Atkins?

Put simply, stop fearing calories!

Take in your fat, restrict your carbs to a reasonable level, and exercise as it makes you feel good, but don't worry too much about exercise right now.

It's been shown that diet trumps exercise in terms of giving us the power to change the way our bodies look, feel, and function, from the inside out. (15)

It is empowering to know that all of that obsession with calorie counting can be let go once and for all.

Calorie restriction isn't the answer anymore, in fact it never was, but we just didn't know it back in the day.

Besides, it's far easier to eat to satiety when you are enjoying high fat foods than it is trying to do the same on a high carb diet, where you never seem to be able to get enough food to satisfy. (16)

It might sound weird for a little while, but once you get to see yourself finally losing the extra weight, you will surely appreciate exactly why the Atkins method has so many followers.

This is an approach to losing fat and maintaining a healthy weight that really does work.

Next up: I will be talking about progress and those pesky scales that are probably on your mind. Just as calorie counting isn't an issue, nor is the weighing scale!

6 THE SCALE ISN'T YOUR CONCERN

Before I begin, let me be clear: I know that this chapter is going to upset some.

If you've been overweight for a good many years, the scale numbers are probably on your mind – constantly!

I'm not saying you shouldn't ever get on a set of scales, but you do need view them less seriously.

A lot of people tend to become obsessed with what those little numbers read.

But those three numbers do not determine your worth as a human being.

You're incredible, just the way you are.

If you want to lose weight in a healthy manner, you have to have a balanced body to go with that balanced mind.

You just have to look at how things are going to go before you get too worked up about everything else.

In other words, you need to make sure that you're looking at your adherence to the different phases of the Atkins diet.

Have you started induction?

Have you gotten through the dreaded low carb flu as explained in chapter four?

Have you decided that you're going to fully commit to this way of eating?

Are you skipping over the high carb foods that moved you away from your weight goal in the first place?

If you haven't yet grasped and adhered to these points, then you have a lot of other things to think about than just the numbers on the scale.

It's all about taking responsibility for your own weight loss journey.

Giving into despair does nothing to get you any closer to your goals, so why panic?

You also need to make sure that you're aware of the different factors that can affect your scale weight to begin with.

The most important thing is that you weigh in at exactly the same time every single day.

If you want to weigh yourself after your first visit to the bathroom in the morning, then you definitely need to make sure you always do this.

It should become a set routine, pretty much like taking your temperature at the same time each day as an accurate way to track your general thyroid function and health.

You also need to realize that if you've taken in a lot of water, that water weight will show up on the scale.

You have to wait till you've passed that fluid out of your system in order to see get an accurate reading. (17)

Don't become discouraged if the weight doesn't appear to be going down, or not moving as fast as you had hoped. Remember, you may still be losing inches.

Unless you get a measuring tape and track all of your bodily changes, you aren't going to really know what you're losing just by the numbers on the scales.

Other indications of progress may show up in the following: Are your clothes fitting better, less tight perhaps?

Do you feel physically and emotionally better than you've felt in a long time?

These factors play a strong role in how likely it is that you will stick to the Atkins diet.

So don't give up before you really get going; wait to see all of the benefits materialize by allowing time for the diet to manifest into your life.

You're worth the effort; you just need to tell yourself this on a daily basis. (18)

Remember too, that weight loss really isn't a simple, straightforward method.

Progress can vary between individuals, meaning sometimes we have to tweak things slightly so as to customize our program to suit our body and needs specifically.

You can't just look at diet as X number of weeks equals Y amount of pounds lost.

It doesn't work that way because your metabolism, your sleep patterns, your food intake, your lifestyle, and your stress levels, all play a part in individual progress. (19)

Next up: I will be talking about one of the key points of concern that many newcomers have: The FAT intake

7 HIGH FAT INTAKE AND WHY FAT IS GLORIOUS

There are so many benefits to be had from dietary fat, but they have been covered up by numerous misconceptions.

I will be the first to admit that when I started on the Atkins diet, I too had my doubts about whether a high fat diet would really be the answer that I was looking for.

I had grown up being told that fat clogged my arteries and how it would increase my risk of heart attack and stroke later on in life.

Even though I don't have any family history of cardiovascular disease, I still didn't want to take my chances, so I did a little research of my own!

I discovered that saturated fat can actually have a very protective effect inside the body. Saturated fat helps to make the hormones necessary for keeping the body running optimally, as well as keeping us fuller for longer after meals.

If you are fed up with constantly snacking all throughout the day, then you definitely need to look into a low carb approach like the Atkins. [20] [21]

The truth is that fat gives us energy.

This is especially noticeable if you're in the Induction phase of Atkins, where your body will primarily run on ketones.

Even the brain has no problem switching over to running on ketones, and in actual fact, it actually becomes even more efficient! (22)

Inflammation is one of the key concerns most folks worry about when it comes to fat intake, though that's not caused by fat at all.

It's actually caused by other complex factors far removed from fat intake.

Stress can be a key driver of inflammation in the body as well, yet it's not brought up nearly as much.

Since foods high in fat are often high in dietary cholesterol, this does give some cause for concern among dieters new to Atkins: what if you're raising your LDL cholesterol to dangerously high levels?

Well, the truth is that the cholesterol you eat doesn't play a role in blood cholesterol levels.

If anything, dietary cholesterol is now linked to improving the "good" blood cholesterol known as high density lipoprotein or HDL.

Low-density lipoprotein (LDL) is the "bad" blood cholesterol, yet this is left unchanged or even slightly lowered with the consumption of foods high in dietary cholesterol.

Worried about strokes? I have friends that are incredibly worried about strokes, and for good reason, they've had to care for family members stricken with this disease.

There is actually a study that was published in the American Journal of Clinical Nutrition in October 2010, where researchers examined the connection between, not only fat and stroke, but fat and other forms of cardiovascular disease as well as cancer risks.

It was discovered that there was no increased concern for fat intake against cardiovascular disease.

The myth is officially dead, debunked by real science.

The study focused on actual Japanese men and women (observational study size: 58,000+) who were regularly eating saturated fats yet showed no elevated risk for heart disease of any kind. (23)

So if you're worried senseless about the amount of fat that the Atkins diet calls for, don't be!

You really have nothing to fear. Eat up and embrace better health, one pat of butter at a time.

In the next few chapters, I will be covering the "mechanics" on the different phases of Atkins.

8 THE PHASES OF ATKINS ARE INCREDIBLY IMPORTANT

Unlike some low carb diets, the Atkins approach is just that - an approach.

There's a certain order to everything, and adhering to it is not considered optional, not if you really want to reap the rewards of living the Atkins lifestyle.

Now, that doesn't mean you're going to be trapped into a system that doesn't serve you, or deprives you in any way.

There are ways to customize the diet to meet your specific needs and without losing any of the benefits.

However, as a newcomer to the approach, I would suggest doing it as "by the book" as possible.

My Atkins book of reference has always been Dr. Atkins New Diet Revolution.

Although this is "older" than the new Atkins publications, I do feel that it sticks to the purity and simplicity of the protocol the best.

OK, so there are basically four phases:
- Phase One: Induction
- Phase Two: Ongoing Weight Loss

- Phase Three: Pre-Maintenance
- Phase Four: Maintenance

By the time you get to phase four – the maintenance phase - you should then be aware of just how many carbs you need in order to maintain the weight goal that you have achieved.

At this point, your carbs may still be lower than what the USDA calls for (300/g/day), but that doesn't mean you're going to have to increase your intake and disrupt your progress.

This should be a phase where you pretty much know what you can eat, what you cannot eat, and how to stay on track.

If you are still struggling at this point, then you may need to go "down" a phase and fine tune your approach. (24)

Don't get discouraged or feel that you need to be on a certain phase for only a short period of time.

There are people who have to be on induction for months in order to correct years, and years of insulin resistance and blood sugar levels that were allowed to run amok.

If you try to pressure yourself, you will only get stressed out, and with stress comes a feeling of pessimism, and the mind will try to convince you, you can't accomplish anything.

You just need to make sure that you're thinking about the bigger picture and pick up from there. (25) (26)

I gave up worrying about what the scales read a long time ago, thanks to the healing power gotten from this way of eating.

It has truly become a positive lifestyle change for me, and I have no doubt that it will eventually become a lifestyle change for you as well.

Check it out. Let yourself go with the flow.

Think only of the benefits that Atkins can deliver into your life.

Develop this mindset and you are bound to reap what so many other followers of this approach have gained.

It can be a bit daunting for a newcomer, but that doesn't have to become an excuse for procrastinating.

Check it out today.

You'll be glad you did!

Next up: I will cover a few more things that you need to know about Phase One, Induction. Yes, that's right, we're revisiting the start, but for good reason.

9 INDUCTION, RELOADED

Some people say that induction is optional, while others will tell you they wouldn't have succeeded without this phase.

They love the way it makes them feel, and they want to experience it for the rest of their lives.

While you might not be thinking that extreme, one thing is clear: there are some benefits derived from induction for everyone.

If you're finding that too many carbs make you sluggish, give induction an honest try.

While it's too "hardcore' for some, the reality is that the induction phase helps you to lose weight like none other.

Instead of running on glucose, the body switches over to burning fat for energy, turning you into a real furnace of dynamism.

There's nothing wrong with staying on induction for a while, or even moving on if you feel the time it right. (27)

I wanted to touch on induction again because a lot of people were saying that it didn't really work for them, and that they found themselves unable to lose weight during this phase.

Maybe you have read accounts of people who claim to actually gain weight while on induction?

For these reasons, there are a few points that I want to raise here with you.

First and foremost, you need to make sure that you're tracking your carbs as much as possible.

You should either buy a carb counting book, or look up everything online.

Don't worry, this isn't a life-long process, as you will surely get to know what's what as you become familiar with the diet and the foods you eat.

For now, you need to know where you stand in terms of carbs intake.

Making sure you're doing what you need to do in order to get where you want to go, is the right approach.

What's important here is that you don't leave anything to guess work.

If you need to lower your carbs, go ahead and lower them.

On the other hand, if you need to raise your carbs, then you should to go ahead and raise them once you leave induction. (28)

As far as induction goes, it's going to be much more important to handle your fat intake properly.

A lot of people think that they're getting enough fat, only to find that they really not.

This is the reason why it's so hard to actually get results on induction.

People try to just "wing it" so to speak, and hope for the best.

It is my opinion that you should not only be tracking your progress, but also be willing to consume a really high amount of fat, that being at least 70% of all of your total calories.

When I was on induction, I was averaging around 80% of fat and without experiencing much stress at all.

In actual fact, it felt wonderful to be able to eat a lot of fat content without worrying about gaining weight.

I left induction soon after I got my weight loss journey jump started.

Induction was pleasant because rather than feeling like I was going to faint if I didn't eat, I could easily go longer between meals without experiencing any shakiness or discomfort.

If you're someone who has the same problem, I would suggest staying in induction for a while to see just how good it can make you feel. (29)

Up next: I will be talking about moving on to Phase Two, Ongoing Weight Loss.

10 PHASE TWO, ONGOING WEIGHT LOSS

If you are looking at trying to lose weight but want to do so in a more controlled fashion, then Phase Two, Ongoing Weight Loss, is exactly where you need to be.

Some people want a little more freedom with food than what Induction allows them, and that means it's time to move up to the next phase.

Keep in mind that if things don't go the way you expected, you can always go back to Induction.

There's nothing in the plan that says that you have to automatically progress to Phase Three if that's not what you want to do.

You just have to make sure that you're thinking ahead in terms of getting things done.

There is something gratifying about being able to say you get to eat a wide variety of food on a low carb diet.

However, you also need to make sure that you have plenty of veggies in your meal plans throughout the week, as this helps to liven up the plate and prevent you from becoming bored with your meals.

What I like to do is set aside a day to actually cook everything that I want to eat for the rest of the week.

If you turn to things like soups, stews, and casseroles, then this approach is actually very doable.

You will be able to just slide out a portion of what you desire and warm it up on the stove or in the microwave oven.

That's really all you have to do in order to make sure you stay on target with your goals.

I always suggest preparing meals ahead of time so that you have plenty of options that are on the plan.

Most people tend to slip off the plan when they aren't paying attention to what's in their fridge or stocked in the cupboards.

When this happens, it's easy to become frustrated because there isn't anything prepared.

This makes it easy to call up the pizza place down the street, even though you know there's no readymade low carb pizza to be had.

So what does Phase Two (Ongoing Weight Loss or OWL) really look like? Let's find out.

Ongoing Weight Loss is a great way to feel like you are taking control over your diet.

There are a few set rules in place which are there to help you keep on track, but mostly, this phase is all about your personal tastes in food.

You will start your first week of OWL at 25 grams of carbohydrates a day, which should still result in you losing weight.

If it doesn't, then you need to make sure that you go back to the drawing board with Induction, until you're ready to start on OWL again.

Sometimes that happens, but for the most part you should still experience weight loss by consuming 25 grams worth of carbs each day.

Be sure that you are thinking carefully about where you want your carbs to come from.

Veggies are by far the best source, but if you prefer fruit or dairy, then that's okay too.

Remember that milk has carbs in it, though cheese has a very low carb count.

That doesn't mean you can go crazy with cheese, but it does give you the freedom to use it for flavoring quite a few low carb dishes. (30)

The special part of OWL comes from the fact that you add in five net carbs per week, providing you are still losing weight, of course.

This is where you might want to get the scales out to help monitor your progress.

I did mean what I said in chapter six about not obsessing about scale weight though.

You need to realize that it's just a tool in the greater scheme of things, and not the be all and end all of tracking your progress. (31)

Another important thing to realize is that the strict Atkins approach does permit you to eat up to 50 grams worth of carbs a day as long as your weight loss isn't stalled.

That really does open the door for some fresh fruit, and even a serving of starchy tubers at dinner, if that's what you want.

Who said this way of eating had to be restricted to boring levels? (32)

Next up: I will cover Phase Three which is all about pre-Maintenance!

11 PHASE THREE, PRE-MAINTENANCE

So, if you've made it this far through the book, then I'm pretty sure you are feeling quite good about committing to the Atkins way of life, right?

Then again, you may still feel a little uneasy at times, especially if some friends and family are not in your corner on this.

There are thousands upon thousands of success stories online which should convince you that this diet really is the way to go.

I am looking forward to going through this chapter with you because it is the phase of Atkins that everyone eagerly awaits, as you're about to find out why.

This is phase three, otherwise known as Pre-Maintenance (PM). PM is a special part of the diet where you get to look at how you've been doing so far.

You should be pretty close to your goal now and only have about 10 pounds left to go.

Instead of adding five grams of daily carbs a week to your diet, the way you did in OWL, this time you're going to bump it up to 10.

...nis won't hinder your progress as you close to your target weight by now.

...ou were at say, 50 grams before adding an ..., it only means you're at 60 g now.

...s increase will give you more food choices, thus ...ing to make it even easier sticking with the program.

Unlike other low carb diets, that usually devolve into a lot of guesswork when things go wrong, you aren't going to face that dilemma here.

The truth is that we are all different, and that means it is you who gets to determine your ideal carb balance, and not some broad theory as set down by so called experts in a publication.

If you are finding that the number in the weighing scales is still not moving in the right direction, then you definitely know that it's because you're taking in too many carbs.

The solution here is to cut back a little and see if that jump starts your weight loss.

If it does, and it's my guess it will do, then you know that the previous limit was simply too much – for you personally - and so you just need to take note and continue on with the program. (33)

If you are trying to add in more foods to your diet, make sure you introduce just one type of food at a time.

If you have cut out diary, then this is the time to add it back and see how you feel.

The same applies to oats or rice.

A serving of rice may not do any harm, but you do need to make sure that you are still tracking your food consumption properly.

The key here is getting to know how your body responds to the various types of food, and once you do, you will soon be preparing your meals without giving it a second thought.

This is a phase that I struggled with.

Once I got the proverbial "green light" to start adding carbs back in, it felt like I was free to do pretty much as I pleased, but I was wrong.

Remember, you're still going to be eating well below what the USDA recommends in terms of carbohydrates. (34)

One thing that I do like about "stepping up" is that you're not just flooding the body with a lot of carbohydrates all in one go.

You are learning how to portion again, something which is essential to eating healthily.

A lot of food and nutritional experts agree that a major contributory factor of global obesity is that our portions have gotten completely out of control. (35)

I think that the obesity epidemic it's a combination of several things.

It's incredibly hard to determine what the root cause actually is, and it's too easy to just say we need to eat less and move more, although eating too much and living sedentary lifestyles is obviously a part of the problem.

The reality is that obesity has a lot of different pathways.

Some people gain weight through hormonal imbalances, while others do it by eating all of the wrong foods.

It would be, in my mind, be incredibly disrespectful to simply assume that everyone who is overweight has reached that point through one "way" above all others.

I'd rather encourage you to embrace the Atkins program as a total lifestyle shift, and let it help you to discover how your body reacts to the foods you eat.

Up next: I am going to cover Phase Four, the "Maintenance" phase, and take a look at what it really means to "maintain" on Atkins?

12 PHASE FOUR IS MORE INTENSE

Maintenance is something that every Atkins follower strives for.

It means that you've reached your target weight, and now you need to retain it once and for all.

I remember when I first reached my own goal and how it felt as though a massive weight had been lifted from my shoulders.

You will probably feel the same way, although your level or elation will depend on how long your journey has taken.

If you are someone who has a hormonal imbalance, then it may take you considerably longer to reach this phase than those who don't have this problem.

Remember, this isn't a sprint, it's a marathon.

It's important that you don't compare yourself to others who have lost more weight in a shorter space of time because you will never get anywhere by doing that.

Trust me, I know all about beating myself up.

I'm still heavily involved in soccer, from being a coach all the way up to still playing a few games.

Am I ever going to be a big time professional?

Nope!

Does that mean that I feel like a lesser person because I'm not Pele?

Not at all! (36)

OK, so let us now look at Phase Four in more detail, and ascertain what it really means for you at this stage of your Atkins journey.

As I said before, Phase Four is all about your goal weight. If you've made it to your goal, you should be feeling very good about yourself by now and quite rightly so.

By the time you reach this phase, you shouldn't be going through any of those ups and downs anymore, or the cravings for foods you missed at the start of your journey.

You should have a lot of your food cravings addressed already if you're moving into Phase Four.

While you can increase your carbs again, it's important to be mindful of the fact that there's more to it now than just watching carbohydrates.

You need to take stock of your current energy levels, as well as the portions that you're consuming.

Ask yourself the following questions:

Am I feeling physically and emotionally better about myself?

Do I finally get to participate in those activities I once had to pass on because I couldn't lose enough weight to partake? (37)

It must stress again: you must make sure you are treating this as a lifestyle change, and not something you can merely stop once you've reached your goals.

It is lifestyle what is going to help you maintain your ideal weight.

There will be occasions when those around you will say you can't do it.

You may get questioned, or criticized even, at family dinner parties about all of the stuff you eat on Atkins.

It can take some getting used to, but don't let other's put you off.

By going through all of the phases of Atkins, you will have learned what you and you alone can and cannot eat; something most other people don't know about themselves!

Even Dr. Atkins himself said that it's no business of others what someone else's body can tolerate with regards to the consumption of food and beverage.

That's a pretty powerful thought, and I think it highlights a bright future ahead as you move into Phase 4. (38)

Up next: I am going to talk about food intolerances, and what it is that makes food intolerances such a problem for some of us?

If you've always wanted to know how to make the Atkins diet work by cutting out or cutting down on certain foods, then this is definitely going to be the best chapter for you!

13 FOOD INTOLERANCES

Food intolerance is not quite the same as food allergies, which is why it doesn't get the same amount of attention.

After all, gluten sensitivity isn't really on the same level as a deadly allergic reaction to shrimp, for example.

I have a friend who's absolutely allergic to peanuts.

It is no laughing matter, although someone we knew thought that he was just trying to get out of sampling her food.

Just a tiny bit of peanut hidden in another dish actually lead to a case of anaphylaxis shock, which is something that is truly life threatening.

Thankfully, my friend carried an epi-pen to counter the reaction, but I still had to go to the hospital with him. (39)

For the rest of us, there are food intolerances.

There's a distinct difference between intolerance to food and an allergy to it.

However, food intolerance is going to be a lot more serious than food sensitivity, although a lot less serious than a true food allergy, where the entire immune system is involved.

If you have an allergy to peanuts, then you can't just have a little serving to avoid the problem.

But if you're gluten intolerant, you may be able to eat a little bread in moderation and still be okay. (40)

However, don't think that there aren't going to be other problems lurking under the surface if you're actually intolerant to a food. For example, a food-intolerance can stall weight loss and cause the body to become inflamed.

When the body is in a constant state of inflammation, it makes it incredibly difficult to lose weight in the way you had hoped. You just have to make sure that you're focusing on what really counts here: your progress.

Whether it's fast or slow, it's still forward, and it's still progress, and that's what matters. (41)

I know it can be difficult to figure out what's really going to affect you as you go through the different phases of Atkins.

You might find that you have to remove foods from your diet one at a time, which is essentially what's happening when working through the different phases.

If you look carefully at the way each phase is set up, you can see that you have to basically add foods back in that are known for causing certain problems within some people.

If you're not someone who responds well to oats, for example, then you can just leave them out of say, Phase Three.

It's all about finding out which foods are going to cause weight gain, which are going to contribute to fatigue, and which are your own personal "power foods" that will keep you feeling as good as possible for as long as possible.

That's the name of the game here, so make sure that you keep working hard at achieving and maintaining your goals.

Up next: I am going to be talking about protein.

More specifically, I want to address the concerns that people have, such as whether or not Atkins is simply a high protein diet. You may be surprised at what you discover!

14 HIGH PROTEIN INTAKE AND THE ATKINS APPROACH

Protein is something that we literally cannot live without.

Being a soccer player, trainer, and a coach, means I'm a huge fan of protein.

Nevertheless, protein tends to be one of the first concerns that people talk to me about when it comes to the Atkins diet.

They wonder how on earth they're ever going to consume the high levels of protein that this diet supposedly calls for. (42)

The thing to be mindful of here is accurate tracking. You should be able to look at solid data that tells you how much protein you're taking in.

Atkins is, first and foremost, more of a high fat diet than a high protein one – right?

This misconception is pretty popular, to the point where people refer to Atkins as the "bacon and steak" diet.

That couldn't be further from the truth.

I don't speak for everyone who has followed Atkins, but I can say that when I do it, it's based on a lot more than just bacon.

I take in good, healthy fats, along with meats and selections in veggies.

I also add in eggs, fish, and even fruit. It's all about looking at where you're at, where your goals are, and what you really want to accomplish.

Sure there are some bodybuilders out there that claim you need a lot of protein in order to build muscle.

However, most people reading this probably don't want to be a bodybuilder at all!

They just want to improve their health and the way in which they look, feel, and function. (43)

Another reason to avoid high amounts of protein is by realizing that any excess gets turned into glucose by the body.

This is why people can consume high levels of meat and still find that they are raising their blood sugar.

This is why there's a time and a place for veggies, and even fruits, on the Atkins approach, depending what Phase you're in.

If you're in Atkins induction, Phase One, then you might feel that you need to limit yourself a bit.

However, you can get lower protein sources like shrimp and various seeds and nuts as a way of having a much more diverse eating plan. (44)

Up next: I will be looking at concerns regarding the Atkins approach and kidney problems.

These are some pretty serious issues, so I know you will want to check out the next chapter to see what it's all about.

15 KIDNEY PROBLEMS AND THE ATKINS APPROACH

You know, I really love covering all the different issues people want addressed with regards to living the Atkins way of life.

Some are worried about not having enough carbs, others are thinking that carbs are completely unnecessary, and plenty more are concerned about serious health problems.

One health problem that immediately comes to mind is the kidney concern.

A lot of people feel that Atkins is a high protein approach to weight loss, and that's just not true.

Protecting the kidneys is crucially important because the body really can't function without them.

In a nutshell, the kidneys are designed to filter out waste products from the blood, as well as excess water.

This then becomes urine, which in turn flows to the bladder where it then gets removed from the body once full.

Your body knows exactly what it's doing with the kidneys.

They are indeed vital organs, even though you can technically still function with diminished kidney performance. (45)

Despite all the talk on this, the truth is that there's no established link between kidney problems and a low carb diet.

This includes concerns with kidney stones as well, something that everyone dreads coming down with.

Kidney stones are incredibly painful, and they can take some time to pass through the system.

There isn't too much doctors can do about Kidney stones except allow them to pass naturally if they are small enough, or remove them through surgery as a last resort.

There was a study published in May of 2012 in the Clinical Journal of the American Society of Nephrology (CJASN), which immediately caught my attention, not least because CJASN is a pretty important medical journal.

I make that distinction because sometimes people question the authority of a study.

If it's good enough to be published in such a prestigious journal, then I definitely want to highlight its findings here for all you readers.

The study focused on not just whether or not a low carb approach like Atkins would be effective, but how it compared to a low-fat approach.

I think that strengthens the nature of this study because it gives you not only an opposite group to measure, but a controlled group as well.

The subjects of the study were examined over the course of four years, and the number of subjects was fairly large for a study of this type: 307!

These partakers were actual humans and not mice or other animals which are raised in labs for medical research.

The participants were fed an actual low carb diet as well.

Although the study doesn't reference pure Atkins with phases and steps, the detailed measurements are pretty important nonetheless.

The result was that there were no harmful effects on kidney function at all, none!

The study did indicate that further research would be necessary before long term conclusions could be drawn, but I'm feeling better already. (46)

Up next: I am going to be talking about sweeteners.

Yes, you can enjoy sweeteners on Atkins, but you need to think carefully about which ones are right and those that should be avoided.

16 SWEETENERS

I couldn't start this chapter on sweeteners if I wasn't willing to talk about sugar.

Sugar is linked to a whole host of health problems.

If you want to embrace a truly low carb lifestyle based on the Atkins approach, then you have to be willing to get rid of sugar from your diet.

This means you have to be conscious of white table sugar, and also be aware of high fructose corn syrup too.

You can't load up on all of those carby sodas if you want to lose weight for the long term.

So you really do need to look at a better alternative sweetener for your Atkins lifestyle. (47)

There are plenty of different sweeteners out there for you to try but they are not all equal or suitable.

You will want to avoid agave, as it is very high in carbohydrates and has a deep impact on blood sugar.

You also want to avoid other forms of sugar, such as honey and maple syrup.

Those sugars just pack on too many carbs to your daily intake, and that's not what we're looking for at all.

Better sources for sweeteners would be xylitol, erythritol, stevia, Splenda (sucralose), and maltitol.

Be careful with the maltitol though as it can cause digestive issues if you consume too much of it! (48)

I think that sweeteners do have their place in Atkins.

We're not going to deny ourselves the sweet taste, so we might as well figure out how to work it in.

I'm not a big fan of dessert myself, but from time to time I do enjoy it and wouldn't like to miss out on such treats.

Remember that if you're using fruit, you really don't need to include a sweetener too.

Let the natural sweetness of the fruit sweeten the dish.

If you're going to be taking in the carbs anyway, then you may as well be served right by them.

Well, that's definitely the idea!

When I first went on Atkins with a friend, we were both surprised at just how hard these sugar cravings could actually be.

If you are someone who is prone to sugar cravings when using sweeteners, then you might want to try going without them for a while.

There is always time to up your intake of coconut oil, which is a healthy fat that can reduce sugar cravings quickly.

Other people like to turn to apple cider vinegar.

Your mileage may vary, so make sure you choose well.

Up next: In chapter 17 I talk about packaged.

It's an important subject, and one of the things that newcomers to Atkins tend to get very wrong.

17 PACKAGED SHAKES, BARS, AND MEALS

This is a touchy issue, so let me be clear: I'm not saying that everyone who goes on Atkins should get into packaged foods, and nor am I suggesting they be avoided.

It's really a mix here, and all about finding the right balance – for you!

The original Atkins approach from 1972 didn't demand that you go with shakes and bars, but other versions of the plan have allowed for them.

After Dr. Atkins passed away in 2003, the company decided to roll out even more Atkins-approved bars, cookies, shakes, and other "treats" designed specifically to keep you on the plan.

Here's the thing: while I think that these items are "legal" in terms of the laws of Atkins, I do feel that they are against the spirit of the diet.

Although we're not counting calories, the same thoughts apply. Liquid carbs (even low counts) tend to be ignored by our minds, in much the same way that liquid calories are for calorie counters.

When we throw everything into a glass, we often don't realize just how much we're taking in.

This neglectful mindset can be dangerous, and as such it should be avoided as much as possible. (49)

Whole foods have a better role in diet, they tend to supply us with the nutrients we need, when we need them.

Trying to get everything from processed shakes and other forms of nutrition is fine if you're on the go, but you really want to let whole foods reign as much as possible.

Again, this is the way it was outlined by Dr. Atkins in 1972. It's a pure approach, but it's one that works and works well.

Obviously I'm not going to sit here and tell you that I don't indulge in a few conveniences here and there, because

I do. It's just that I do so in a different way.

I like to take a cooler when I'm going to be on a trip for a while, and I also believe in packing the most convenient whole foods that I can get.

There's absolutely nothing wrong with using jerky as a snack when you're surrounded by the siren song of high carb goodies everywhere. (50)

By now you should know exactly what you need to do to rock an Atkins template.

If you're lost at this point, go back and check the chapters on all of the Phases of Atkins.

You may even have to go back to Induction, where sweeteners are actually not allowed, and you will need to cut out the processed stuff as well.

However, there is so much power found in freeing yourself from that type of thing, really!

Up next: Here I am going to cover a topic that doesn't get mentioned all that much: appetite control!

Hormones are involved in how hungry we feel; something that most people don't realize.

In the next chapter I will break it down for you so that you don't have to stress about being Atkins compliant!

18 APPETITE CONTROL

So, I take it by now that you have read up on all of the phases of Atkins and that you're feeling more confident than ever?

I'm so glad.

But now is not the time to rest on your laurels as there are many other parts of the diet yet to cover.

You see, not everyone has a good time on Atkins.

And those who don't, start wondering if they are ever going to lose weight and truly feel great, as has been promised to those who truly embrace the Atkins way of life.

The reality here is that you can't just assume everything is going to line up easily and without the need for a little tweaking.

We humans are different to one another in various ways.

What helps me to lose weight might not work for you at all, or may even contribute towards weight gain in your case.

While I'm confident that Atkins is a great approach for everyone, I will admit that there can be glitches along the way.

No all the time, and not with every individual, but setbacks can and do happen sometimes with some people.

One problem is definitely that of appetite control.

If you're constantly feeling hungry then you're going to address that hunger by consuming food.

There's just no other way around it. Once you get into the food mindset, that's where you're going to be for a while.

Many hardline dieters will say that you should just grit your teeth and get through it the best way you can.

However, I think there are forces at play here that you should know about.

For example, did you know that the protein hormone leptin plays a strong role in how hungry we feel?

If you're not familiar with leptin, then allow me to tell you all about it.

You see, leptin is one of the main hormones responsible for telling the brain when it's time to eat, that is, we feel hungry.

Leptin is actually in the fat tissues themselves, and overweight people generally have sky-high levels of this master hormone.

However, the way in which leptin functions is not always accurate. In some cases, it's possible for the body to be leptin resistant.

What this means to a person who is leptin resistant is that they never truly feel full even though they've actually eaten ample amounts. (51)

There have been studies conducted on leptin, as well as on energy balance for research into ways of addressing obesity.

A study published in the Proceedings of the National Academy of Sciences of the United States of America (April 2001), indicates that if we address leptin, we can in turn address stubborn weight, that is, those excess pounds that just will not shift no matter what. (52)

Addressing leptin resistance is not something that can be tackled overnight.

Diet, exercise, sleep, and stress management, all play a strong role in how well leptin regulates in the body.

This means that in order to get the best results from a change in diet and pursue a positive lifestyle change, you are going to have to go to bed at a reasonable hour.

It also means you will have to work at getting stress levels down, if indeed stress is an issue in your life.

I'm a big supporter of getting out of the "busy, busy, busy" lifestyle.

I think it's one of the key factors in why the obesity epidemic has gotten so out of control.

The more stress we have in our lives, the more the body thinks it has to hang on to every ounce of fat we have.

This isn't a new conclusion, but it's one we humans choose to ignore all the time.

You are not Superman, or woman, so there's no need to fly around trying to fix the world's problems. (53)

Eating properly and lowering your carbohydrate count, as per the Atkins Nutritional Approach, is definitely the way to go.

This addresses your hormone health on the inside, and your weight loss issues on the out.

What more could you ask for in an eating plan?

Up next: I will cover a social problem that many experience when joining the Atkins program: "Dining Out."

If you are tired of hiding indoors just because you started on Atkins, then it's time to get you out again.

In the next chapter I will give you some food for thought and show you how it's quite possible to remain socially active without going off plan!

19 DINING OUT

I remember when I first joined Atkins. I did it "strict style", which meant I started at the Atkins Induction phase.

It was definitely a wakeup call on a number of levels.

Firstly, it highlighted to me how sugar consumption was way, way, out of control, and a major contributor to the obesity epidemic.

I gave up bread and soon realized how much it had been holding me back.

I wanted a vibrant, healthy existence, and knew I could achieve it so long as I never forgot how the regular way of eating had been responsible for blocking me at every turn.

However, I also wanted to be social and hang out with friends.

I didn't want to give up doing certain things or going to places that I enjoyed pre-Atkins.

Sometimes we become so worried about going "off plan" that we tend to shut people out of our lives that we really don't want to exclude.

I was also married by the time I began living the Atkins way, and my wife certainly had no plans for us to stay home forever just because my eating habits had changed!

So this got me thinking.

If you're on Atkins right now, it really depends on what phase you're at.

And it's my guess that you are really glad you don't have to count calories, only carbs?

I found a study which showed that calorie counting restaurant foods may be way off the chart anyway.

This means, for the calories conscious dieter, overeating can definitely be problematic when eating out.

Even though your main focus is to count carbs, I do find that calories have an interesting role in our overall health nonetheless.

You want to stick to nutrient dense food as much as possible.

Skipping those breaded appetizers will definitely be part of what keeps you on track. (54)

From here on, you definitely need to start getting comfortable with speaking up about what you're going to eat and what you're not going to eat.

A lot of people think that they are being rude when they tell servers what to leave off of their plates, but that doesn't make sense at all.

You are the paying customer and as such you should be getting your own way within reason.

As long as you're polite, I don't see what's so wrong with making sure you're getting exactly what you are prepared to pay for.

This might mean skipping the toast and ordering more vegetables, but so be it.

Vegetables are so much more Atkins-friendly anyway, and it's not as if you asking for something that isn't on the menu.

Loading up on the veggies and getting in some good protein will leave you feeling fuller for longer.

If you are dining at a restaurant where they can bring you some butter; then feel free to ask for extra.

Remember, Atkins i̇ͅ
rather than a truly high-proᴛ̣

Being mindful of this ma̤
eating out.

Breakfast should be pretty easy.
like a big plate of bacon and eggs?

If you want to do fruit, I would go
berries because they are fairly low in terms o̤

The tart taste of blueberries is something   ͺok
forward to all the time.

Keep in mind that as people start seeing how healthy and vibrant you look, they're going to ask you to share your secret.

You already know about the power of leptin in your overall health, but you also can speak to them confidently about your Atkins way of life. (55)

Up next: I am going to be covering sugar cravings.

This is yet another key problem that many Atkins followers talk about early on.

The last thing I want is for you to become derailed by stumbling on this common setback, so definitely check out the next chapter.

20 SUGAR CRAVINGS

I talked a little about the problems with sugar in Chapter 16, but I figured we needed to dig a little deeper into the topic at this point.

Sugar is pretty addictive, and we finally have the science to back something up that we've been talking about for a long time in nutrition circles.

You see, a study published in June of 2013, over at the American Journal of Clinical Nutrition, indicates that high-sugar foods affect reward as well as our cravings.

The study specifically focused on men, but I think there are conclusions that can be made for women here too. (56)

The study has credence because it's not just a "survey" type of research.

It's one that digs directly into the consumption of food. It focused on 12 overweight and/or obese men that consumed meals which were both high on the glycemic index, and low on the GI.

To the researchers, the results were astonishing.

They expected the high GI meals to have minimal effects (something many experts have claimed over time). However, that wasn't the case at all.

What they found is that the high-GI meals increased hunger immensely, going on for some hours.

This had consequences for the next meal, where the over-consumption of food was the after-effect, as a way to curb this "hunger".

Now that we know just how addictive sugar is, how do we really address the problem?

Well, for a start we can increase our fat intake.

Increasing dietary fat has long been considered a way to make us feel fuller for longer, with multiple studies drawing links between increased lipids and lower food intake from meals later on, after the fat has been in the system. (57), (58), (59), (60)

So, if sugar cravings are an issue with you, then I think you should definitely increase your fat intake.

However, if you're not tracking how much fat you're getting, then there is no way to tell where you started at.

This is why I always emphasize the importance of tracking your food at every opportunity until you hit Phase Four.

The best way to track your food is to do it online.

This way you can simply key it in and then go on with your day.

Sometimes, remembering to stop and write things down on paper is utterly exhausting, and it's the last thing we really want to do if we can help it.

Now is the best time to take stock of your progress. Not just your diet, but also look at how you're feeling overall.

If you are still not feeling as good as you had hoped, then you might need to address your sleep habits as well as your diet.

Everything is connected, but it's a hard lesson to learn.

And even if you are getting enough sleep in terms of hours per night, that doesn't necessarily mean you are getting enough "quality" kip.

Only you will be able to address such questions.

Unfortunately, the media is full of quick fixes, misinformation, and fad diets when it comes to weight loss.

We keep telling people that all they have to do is move more and eat less, or go on some new wonder diet and 'lose 10 pounds in 10 days', after which everything will be just fine and dandy.

I think that the solution to weight loss is much more complex than this; in fact I know it is.

This is actually why the Atkins Nutritional Approach is structured the way it is.

It's about your life, not just your weight.

In my opinion, that's exactly the right approach to successful weight loss, weight maintenance, and healthy living.

On the topic of fat intake, we are now about to go into healthy fats in the next chapter.

21 HEALTHY FATS

What do you think the best part about a low carb diet is?

For me that's easy. It has to be the increased amount of good, healthy fats you get to eat, but this is where a lot of people still don't quite understand the Atkins approach.

So many continue to assume it's a high-protein diet, when it's really a high fat one. (61)

Before I really dig into the topic of healthy fats, let me first ease some of your concerns.

One of the common misconceptions newcomers make is by thinking the high consumption of extra fat in a regular diet is bound to see them keel over sooner rather than later.

Well, just know that this is not the case at all.

If anything, there is more of an indication now on how sugar contributes towards poor heart health than dietary fat ever did.

This isn't news actually. There was a study done by John Yudkin way back in May 1978 that confirmed this.

Unfortunately, the scientific community dismissed these findings completely, opting instead to jump on the saturated fat bandwagon; telling consumers that this was the real villain in the story. (62)

If you're going to go with healthy fats in the diet, then you have to know which ones to avoid and which ones to enjoy.

Personally, I still think avoiding trans-fats is something that you should strive for.

However, I also believe that your diet should fit your lifestyle. If you're on the go, it's very hard to avoid all of those partially hydrogenated oils.

Do what you can, when you can, and whatever you do, don't beat yourself up.

Dr. Atkins told people in many of his books that it's better to do your best and make mistakes, than it is to assume that everything is hopeless.

The latter outlook wouldn't make sense at all, and you shouldn't resign yourself to such thoughts of doom and gloom anyway. (63)

As I go through the Atkins program, I have found that butter, beef fat (tallow), pork fat (lard), olive oil, coconut oil, and even chicken fat, is good.

Obviously you don't have to eat these things with a spoon in order to get sufficient amounts of fat.

I have a few tips that will help you get your fat intake up in a more subtle way:

First and foremost, make sure that you add butter to those soups! It will give them a really rich flavor, plus it doesn't add any carbs.

You can enjoy butter and really bring your fat levels up. Seriously, there is nothing wrong with having a 70% fat day.

There is also an opportunity to cook all of your meals in tallow or lard, which will obviously increase your fat intake.

You can easily deep fry in tallow or lard too.

Pork rinds make a good replacement for bread, and a very low carb one at that.

Adding in bacon and fatty cuts of beef to your meals is another way to increase your fat consumption.

If you feel like drinking your fat, add heavy cream to coffee for a fat punch that's still right on plan.

You will need to modify everything based on which Phase of Atkins you are on, but you're bound to still have good results wherever you're at.

Up next: I am going to address thyroid issues; one of the big issues overlooked by Atkins followers. Read on so you don't make the same mistake!

22 THYROID PROBLEMS

The thyroid is an amazing gland of the human body.

No, seriously, please, hear me out for a minute.

I realize this isn't likely to be a topic for discussion that you thought we'd be having as you're get into living the Atkins lifestyle, but it's an important one nonetheless, so I advise not to skip this section.

It's important that you understand everything the thyroid does in the body.

This way, you are better prepared if you have thyroid issues.

First and foremost it produces hormones which regulate our energy balance.

A thyroid that isn't functioning properly can contribute towards long periods of chronic fatigue.

You may have a hypothyroid, a condition where the body just doesn't produce the right amount of thyroid hormones that it needs, and that can be a real drag! (64)

Iodine supplementation is one of the key ways to improve your thyroid function.

The good news is that this can be done via the Atkins approach.

You just need to make sure that you get the right amount of iodine for your situation.

It's a good idea to first do a test to check whether or not you're deficient in iodine.

If your doctor will not test for you, don't worry.

There are some home kits that you can purchase which allow you to send your samples of to a lab for accurate analysis. (65)

There's also a disorder known as hyperthyroidism.

When this occurs the thyroid is out of control. In this case, you will likely experience weight loss, but that's not as good as you might think.

Hyperthyroidism also creates another problem, and that is you become restless and irritated.

This in turn sends your body and mind off balance, resulting in sleeplessness.

Nervousness and sweating often accompany hyperthyroidism too.

This is not something that you want to ignore.

If you feel that you may need more help than first thought, then it's always a good idea to see your doctor at your earliest possible convenience. (66)

A low carb diet is a great way to reset the body.

Eating low carb meals means you're not as hungry as often, so the body has time to focus on something other than how much food you're consuming.

If you are still unsure about Atkins, but you're fed-up with being tired all the time, then you definitely want to see what this approach to eating can do for you.

It's not all deprivation, as many Atkins fans will attest to. It's all about working with your body in order to have it function at its best.

When it comes down to it total wellness, both inside and out, is really what we're striving towards here.

You don't have to feel like the Atkins approach is an impossible task because it's not, far from it in fact.

Just start with the Atkins Induction (Phase One) and go from there.

If you need to reread the previous chapters about that, including potential issues that can come up with induction, simply go back and read through the relevant pages.

I think that the thyroid controls a lot more than we give it credit for, and it's high time we give it a chance to truly serve our bodies.

Feeding yourself the Atkins way provides you with a lot of fresh, healthy foods, including lots of veggies, which help to nourish the thyroid.

Up next: I am going to look at supplementation options that can really complement the Atkins lifestyle.

23 DON'T IGNORE THE POWER OF POTASSIUM

If you automatically think that reaching for a banana is the only way you're ever going to get all your potassium needs, then think again.

The truth is that bananas raise blood sugar far too much to be useful for us low carb people.

Atkins is just another low carb diet with a tiered approach.

I aim this chapter more towards the newcomer who is not anywhere near Phase Four.

If you're already in Maintenance, then you can enjoy a bit more fruit than someone who isn't there yet.

This doesn't mean that you're at a disadvantage as a newbie.

It just means you have a little further to go in your journey than someone who is at phase four. (67)

So, where do we actually go from here?

Well, you might be surprised at just how many low carb foods are really rich in terms of potassium.

For example, you can have avocado, Swiss chard, yogurt, and even red peppers.

These are all going to be healthier options that have far fewer carbs than bananas do, and they're pretty tasty to boot.

I love having Swiss chard at dinner right next to a big, juicy steak.

Will your mileage vary?

Of course it will.

But I did want to bring this to your attention nonetheless. (68)

Low potassium is a pretty dangerous thing.

It can affect your heart, your energy balance, and cause painful muscle cramps.

I highly doubt that anyone wants to experience unnecessary pain!

This is where you really need to think about the way you are feeling, and get your potassium levels up if necessary.

Low potassium levels can manifest in a number of ways, perhaps most noticeable by feeling tired and run down.

If you are experiencing this then it's important to get your body back into balance as soon as possible.

The best and most direct way of doing this is to first try changing things around in your diet.

The amazing thing about Atkins is that there's so much flexibility, and because we monitor what we eat, it should be pretty easy to make and monitor adjustments in diet.

You don't have to feel as though you are doomed to eat the same things over and over again.

It's just helpful if you follow a similar template as you learn about Atkins, just until such times as you get become really familiar with your program.

Once you are comfortable with all the phases, you will be well on your way to a maintenance lifestyle that you can count on. (69)

Potassium plays an important role in the body from head to toe.

It is really one of those minerals that we can't function without, so you do need to ensure you're getting the amounts your body needs.

It is when we are low on potassium that trouble strikes.

But when we have all that we need, we feel happier, healthier, and balanced overall.

Try peeling an avocado and savor it. There's a good source of both fiber and potassium in that wonderful fruit. (70)

Up next: I will be covering the importance of magnesium, which is another useful mineral that we low carbers need plenty of!

24 DON'T SKIP THE MAGNESIUM

I don't advocate too much supplementation on the Atkins Nutritional Approach.

In my opinion, you should be able to almost anything and everything you need from food alone.

However "almost" is not quite good enough, hence a little help from supplementation - in moderation or course!

Most of us are busy people; such is the way of the world these days.

Sometimes it seems as though we're on the go nonstop.

None of us eat 100% the way that we're supposed to eat, not even the most health-conscious among us.

This means that "some" supplementation has to be in the game plan in order us to sustain the healthy and vibrant lifestyle that we deserve for our efforts.

We can start by adding in more magnesium.

Magnesium regulates a lot of different reactions in the body (over 300 of them).

You can't even manage your own metabolism without the help of magnesium.

Stress acts negatively on the body by attacking stores of magnesium.

If stress is evident in your busy lifestyle then you especially will have to replenish your magnesium holdings each day in order to feel and function right.

Just as we need potassium to avoid painful muscle cramps, we also need plenty of magnesium as well.

The two minerals actually work together, so it's helpful to supplement both. (71), (72)

There are new studies which indicate magnesium is incredibly vital to the human body.

You can actually get magnesium into the body by taking Epsom salt baths.

My wife went Atkins with me to make things easier, and she absolutely loves bathing in Epsom bath salts.

If you're someone who isn't too keen on taking long soaks in the tub, then you can always just soak your feet.

The minerals can still be absorbed just fine with a foot bath. (73)

Magnesium is also found in fish, as well as in leafy greens.

You should be eating your leafy greens anyway, but this just proves how important it is to have a colorful diet, rich with vegetable matter, as much as it is to have protein.

If you're tired of red meat, changing to fish is a good idea.

I don't want anyone to think for a second that you can't do amazing things with low carb eating.

You can fuel your body, have an amazing life, and experience lots of fun along the way.

I just wanted to bring your attention to these highly critical nutrients that the body needs in order to thrive optimally.

Only after we've powered our body can we truly reap the health benefits that we're striving for.

Up next: I will be looking at Vitamin D as part of this mini-series on supplementation.

25 VITAMIN D

In a perfect world, food alone would give us all the nutrition we need, and more besides.

However, the world that we live in is far from perfect.

This means we have to get some of our nutrients from sources other than food if we are to strike the right nutritional balance in our lives.

Getting Vitamin D (cholecalciferol) into your body is not always a simple case of exposing yourself to a little sunlight.

The truth is that the sun doesn't shine the same way everywhere on earth, and in northern Scandinavia, some regions are lucky to see an hour of daylight a day during mid-winter.

And some countries get a lot more dense cloud cover than others.

This is why vitamin D supplementation is well worth consideration.

A Vitamin D deficiency can result in you feeling lethargic.

There are also links between Vitamin D deficiency and depression.

This is why it's important to make sure you get as much as of this essential vitamin as possible, whenever possible. (74)

Aside from sunlight, we can get Vitamin D by consuming more eggs.

It's also found in cod liver oil.

However, you may be better off by taking Vitamin D3 supplements, just to make sure you are getting the required amounts.

This will help keep your levels up even when the sun isn't shining, or you're locked indoors at work during daylight hours.

Some people swear by supplementation as a solution, particularly during the long winter months, and especially if they are affected by Seasonal Affective Disorder, or SAD syndrome.

Keep in mind too, that age and skin color plays a role in how much Vitamin D you're able to get from the sun alone. Younger people tend to get their levels up much better than older people, for example.

And it's been shown that people with darker skin have to stay out in the sun longer than those of a fairer complexion just to absorb the same amounts. (75), (76)

When I get plenty of exposure to sunlight, I feel so much better, both physically and mentally, and I know I'm not alone on that score.

Go out in the sun yourself.

Make sure you don't put on a lot of UVB-blocking sunscreen too because those UVB rays are what trigger your body into manufacturing the Vitamin D that it needs.

You don't have to stay out there all day, yet this is where most people get their information wrong.

They think they have to expose themselves to the sun for extended periods, but this is just plain wrong.

Furthermore, exposing ourselves to long periods of direct sunlight is what damages the skin.

Not only will you age prematurely, but you will also have an increased risk of cancer.

So it's important that you are mindful on the importance of moderate exposure.

You might be wondering how this is directly tied in with the Atkins approach?

Well, if you're going to go on a strict Atkins protocol, then I think it is well worth your time and effort to ensure you are addressing your health as a whole.

Up next: I will be covering calcium; yet another highly important mineral that we can't do without.

26 CALCIUM

So far in this little mini-series on supplementation, I have discussed some key players, namely Vitamin D, potassium, magnesium, and now calcium.

But what is calcium, and more importantly, what's all the fuss about? Let us now find out.

Calcium is a mineral our body needs in order to build strong bones, teeth, and gums. It also helps our nerves carry messages all around the body.

Without calcium, the body would break down very quickly and we'd experience serious health problems as a result. (77)

Both men and women need calcium, obviously! But there has been a lot of focus on calcium in women, given the risk of osteoporosis being higher in females than males.

Even so, both genders really do need to get sufficient calcium into their body. (78)

Some people have spread the myth that an Atkins diet abundant in meat keeps the body from really utilizing calcium efficiently.

Since I just mentioned bone density loss (osteoporosis), you may have some cause for alarm right now.

That's the way myths are designed; to steal progress when you could be enjoying the best weight loss and weight maintenance journey of your life.

There have been numerous studies conducted on this very issue, including one published in the American Journal of Clinical Nutrition in 1983.

The research concluded that a diet higher in protein (including a diet rich in meat) didn't have an effect on calcium metabolism the way it was first predicted (79).

If anything, you should be enjoying a diet rich in protein for its own benefits.

Although Atkins is technically a high fat diet more so than a high protein one, you are still getting all the protein you need every single day (80).

With options available to you such as nuts, cheese, milk, leafy greens, and sunflower seeds, there is no reason at all why you can't get all the calcium you need from food.

However, have you ever considered unlocking the calcium out of your bones?

Did you know, for example, that our ancestors ate most of their meat straight off the bone?

What's more is that these bones were cooked in acidic mediums as a way to make them soft enough to crack open. Getting into the core of the bone gave access to the marrow within.

Calcium would then be along for the ride with that marrow, thus supplying the body with all its nutritional requirements.

Now, I'm not proposing you head off down to the local butcher and order a bag of bones.

But I am suggesting that it might be wise to get a calcium supplement if you find that you're not taking in enough through diet alone.

Up next: I will be looking at iron and the role this essential mineral plays in the body, and how it fits into the Atkins way of living.

27 IRON AND THE ATKINS DIET

Since I already covered potassium, magnesium, calcium and Vitamin D, I figured it would be a good idea to look at iron as well. It's quite amazing just how many different minerals work together to fuel our bodies?

It might sound weird, but I think this part of science is fascinating.

If you have too much of something, you're going to have problems.

But if you have too little of a specific nutrient, then you're also going to have problems.

Therefore, our aim here is balance.

Finding the right balance is something that might be hard to grasp at first, but as this series goes on I think you'll get what I'm saying.

Iron is one of those essential minerals that we simply have to have.

There's plenty written down on how much iron we need, as well as how iron is metabolized by the body.

I read a study published in the Journal of the American Medical Association that indicates the problem of iron deficiency is actually higher than first thought.

Now, this is a study from 1997, but I think it's still pretty relevant today.

We need to get iron into our system, and moreover we need to make sure we're getting it regularly. (1), (2)

So what does iron do exactly?

The answer to that is plenty!

Iron handles the transportation of red blood cells in the body through hemoglobin and myoglobin.

Iron also has a role in other proteins within the body. Given this, it might not be surprising that many sources of protein also give us plenty of iron.

Do you eat eggs for breakfast?

Good. Eggs not only provide you with protein, but they are also a good source of iron too.

The yolk is where most of the iron is, so don't throw out those yolks anymore! (3)

You will also find iron in some dried beans as well as dried fruits.

Stay away from iron-fortified cereals though. In my opinion, they provide way too many carbs so it's just not worth it.

You're better off getting your iron out of red meat, poultry, tuna, salmon, shellfish, and some leafy greens as well.

It has been shown that vegetable sources are a bit tougher for the body to get the iron out of, but this can be made easier by cooking your greens as opposed to eating them raw.

Up next: I will be covering sodium consumption and taking a look at whether that salt is really going to hurt you while enjoying the best that the Atkins Nutritional Approach has to offer?

28 SODIUM INTAKE

I will lead this chapter with an opinion: I don't think that there's any reason in the world to fear salt.

We humans know how important it is in our diet.

We actually have a very long tradition of using salt, which I think is good.

Of course, the salt you choose does actually make a difference.

I prefer sea salt whenever possible. From sea salt you get some good trace minerals which are important.

Furthermore, sea salt tends to be a much more flavorful choice for most people. (84)

Newcomers to Atkins have concerns over sodium, which is why I think we need to address this here.

It's perfectly okay to be concerned about the amount of sodium you're getting.

But you have to realize that when you go on a low carb diet like the Atkins Nutritional Approach, you're changing the way your body functions.

So when you read studies that show health problems associated with salt, you have to look at the way the study was conducted.

If the people highlighted in the research weren't eating the same way that you do, then why would their diet have an effect on you?

It's easy to panic over a headline, but it takes a little more reading to fully understand what these studies are actually telling us.

Don't worry if you've been taken in by a misleading study or two, as most of us have from time to time, including me.

There are some people who are genuinely salt sensitive, to the point where excess sodium plays a role in high blood pressure and bad heart health.

However, most of us are not so sensitive to salt.

We actually need it in order to regulate hormones, handle energy balance, and other things in between. (85)

This is one debate that will rage onwards as such nutritional debates tend to do.

Does this mean I think it's nonsensical to skip the salt?

Of course not!

There are cases where low sodium is absolutely necessary.

If your physician says that you should be taking in less sodium, it's wise to follow doctor's orders – specifically - in order to protect your health.

But there are some studies that have caught my attention.

There was a report published in the European Heart Journal that indicates salt intake and cardiovascular disease (something we all try to avoid) aren't as linked as first thought (86).

Indeed, there is still cause for some concern and there should definitely be continued discussions and further research on salt intake.

But far too many people are just assuming that this means we have to have a super low sodium diet for no apparent reason.

Until the connections are studied at a deeper level, I think that the massive alarm and panic over sodium intake is unwarranted. (87)

Up next: I will be talking about fiber.

If you think fiber isn't just as controversial as sodium intake, then you might want to think again!

29 FIBER AND THE ATKINS DIET

Fiber is an important dietary substance that's good for our health. There, I said it!

A lot of people new to the Atkins Nutritional Approach believe that they just won't get enough fiber in their diet.

You will be pleased to know that this is not the case.

When done correctly, the Atkins diet is balanced enough to give you all of the fiber your body needs, so there's no real need to worry about missing out on your daily roughage.

Fiber actually has a strong role in the body. It can help prevent constipation, ensuring that you're able to evacuate bodily waste without issue.

There's no worse feeling than bowel movements that are hard to pass. There are actually two different types of fiber, namely soluble and insoluble.

Soluble fiber helps to keep cholesterol lower. Psyllium is a source of soluble fiber and something that you can still have on Atkins. You can also enjoy lemon as well.

Carrots are a bit higher in carbs, but you can have those too. Peas and beans are two more very good sources of fiber. (88)

Insoluble fiber is what helps the body to eliminate waste. Cauliflower is chock full of insoluble fiber, and that's a low carb staple.

Fiber has a deep role in the body.

When it comes to something as serious as say coronary heart disease, it can step in to save the day.

A study published by the Journal of the American Medical Association discovered that long term fiber intake can reduce the risk of coronary heart disease in women.

Heart disease is a leading cause of death for women, which means we definitely need to do everything we can to prevent it. If adding more fiber to the diet is part of that prevention, then so be it.

There is a study published in the American Journal of Clinical Nutrition that focused more on starchy carbohydrates for fiber, but I think there's still some wisdom in here for us Atkins people.

Fiber is connected to a decrease in risk for ischemic heart disease.

This study was done in 1972, right around the same time that Dr. Atkins was just getting started on his theories into carb intake. (89)

I think that we have a lot to learn here, and we should never stop learning and adapting. Incorporating fiber into your diet via the Atkins approach is very doable.

Add sugar snaps and snow peas later on as you inch closer towards Phase Four.

Don't forget cucumber, carrots, and cauliflower are all great sources for fiber too (90).

Up next: I will be covering caffeine intake. I know that this can be pretty controversial, but it's important.

I care about my readers and want you to experience the best Atkins journey possible.

Avoiding common mistakes along the way is the key to your continued success.

30 CAFFEINE

Before I begin, let me be clear: I'm a big coffee fan.

I hope my wife isn't reading this because I really do love coffee... a lot.

Not as much as I love my wife, but still!

I don't think that coffee and caffeine has to dominate my life though, and that's the focus of this chapter.

Far too often with Atkins, and other low carb diets, we let caffeine rule over us, instead of us ruling over it.

Let us begin by looking at caffeine and discovering what it's all about.

Many of us simply think that caffeine is coffee, but this is not actually so.

Caffeine is found in other things too, including chocolate, tea, and even some ice creams.

Caffeine is a stimulant that makes us feel more alert.

It's very possible to overdo caffeine to the point where we can't go through our day without feeling the need for those additional java fixes.

Giving up coffee might not sound like something that should be on your list of priorities, but it's incredibly important to control how much you drink.

In fact, I would say it's so important it should be made a priority. (91)

Can you have coffee while you're on Atkins Induction?

Absolutely, but, and it is a big BUT, you need to modify your intake.

If you're aiming for ketosis, then trying to get a load of sweetener into your coffee isn't the answer.

Induction prohibits sweeteners, and it's crucial to follow the plan specifically so as to get on the right track with weight loss journey.

When you really step back and see how the phases blend into each other, you can appreciate all the carefully thought out work that Dr. Atkins put into this way of eating.

It's not simply the "butter and bacon" diet, as some people believe it to be.

Atkins is a blueprint for consistent weight loss and weight maintenance that truly works when followed properly.

Ketosis is powerful because we become fat burners instead of sugar burners, and that has a lot of benefits. (92)

Still, there is a place for caffeine in our world. Personally, I like to take a cup of coffee before my workouts, which leaves me with enough energy to really go for that last set.

Apparently, I'm not the only one. Having a cup of java before working out has become a mini-movement - of sorts – among us fitness types.

If this is you, then you definitely want to make sure you're charged up for a great workout at the gym, and that cup of coffee can work in your favor.

In my opinion, anything that helps folks get into the gym is truly a good thing.

We need more people doing some form or workout along with eating right. (93)

If you are controlling your caffeine intake to sensible levels, then there's nothing wrong with it at all.

But when some of my friends tell me they go through at least 2-3 pots of coffee a day, I find myself being both alarmed and concerned for their health.

A lot of people say they need their caffeine fixes just to stay awake and alert throughout the day.

If this sounds like you, then you owe it to yourself to find the real reason behind why you're so incredibly tired all the time, and not just brush it off with heaps of coffee.

Up next: I am going to be taking a look at alcohol.

31 ALCOHOL ON ATKINS -- WORTH LOOKING INTO

Since I probably upset the die-hard caffeine hounds with the last chapter, I guess I need to kick the hornet's nest here by talking to those of you who love going out for a few drinks after a hard day at work.

Don't get me wrong; when my friends and I are out and about, we have a great time.

However, now that I'm on Atkins, I had to devise a way of having a few drinks without killing my progress.

There are plenty of alcoholic beverages that you can enjoy without upsetting your carb limits.

For example, whiskey, vodka, gin, rum, and tequila, are all incredibly good choices for low carb drinking.

However, beware of the mixers!

Some of the mixers added to these drinks can be incredibly sugary.

If you want to make low carb cocktails, then you are going to need to scan the ingredients carefully before you mix.

You may get a deeper appreciation for alcohol after this journey. After all, you're going to learn more about how alcohol beverages taste without the sugary stuff we add to mask the true flavors.

Enjoying your drinks "neat" is a great way to make sure you're managing your carbs in a more controlled way. (94)

One popular misconception is that alcohol breaks down into sugar.

That's not true at all.

The fact is that the liver is responsible for breaking down alcohol into acetate first. After that, it will be broken down further into CO_2 and water.

Sugar doesn't even come into the equation.

You can actually be in ketosis and drink, but you need to realize that you are going to be burning the alcohol first.

This means that no fat deposits are getting burned to fuel your body. (95)

Obviously there are natural concerns around alcohol consumption, or overconsumption to be more precise.

It would be negligent of me if I failed to point that out.

You should know that if you're having a hard time controlling your consumption of alcohol, then it will much better to give it up altogether than to repeatedly fail to control your drinking.

Obviously what you drink, and how much, is completely up to you and all I can do is advise.

At the end of the day, I feel that drinking is a personal and private decision. If you're okay with drinking in moderation, then you will be fine as it relates to Atkins.

But if you are finding that your consumption is affecting your personal life, then you may want to pull back completely.

As I say, the ball is in your court on this one (96).

Up next: We will be looking at an approach some Atkins followers use to handle stubborn weight loss plateaus:

The Fat Fast!

32 THE FAT FAST

Let's face it, weight loss can be hard for many people, especially if the plan they are on is not right for them personally.

It would be foolish to assume that every single one of my readers will lose weight in exactly the same way.

This is why so much care has been given to each individual chapter.

I want to make sure that you have the keys necessary to unlock your own success.

Moreover, I don't want you to make the same mistakes that I made when first starting out.

There was a period of time where I struggled to lose any weight at all and it was downright awful.

I felt alone in the game and even a little helpless, not knowing quite where to head next.

What made this time particularly frustrating was that I felt as though I was doing every phase perfectly.

I didn't even have cheat days!

And yet I came to a point where I just wasn't able to lose any more weight.

Enter the Atkins Fat Fast. (97)

Now, let me start by saying that this isn't for everyone.

The Fat Fast is four to five days of strict calorie counting, but with foods that are also going to be low carb in nature.

If this is something that's going to be next to impossible for you, you may want to skip it.

However, if you get to feel anywhere near as lost and hopeless as I did, then you will be desperate to see if there's anything that you can possibility do to get things moving in the right direction again.

Here's the thing: you are going to be on about 1000-1200 calories for this five day stretch.

You will want to break this down into five feeds of about 200 calories each, just to give you a little margin for error.

This is a pretty limited diet with about 90% fat. It is actually designed to push you into ketosis.

There's no way that you're going to be able to ignore it either.

You just have grit your teeth and get on with it.

With a strong determination and the will to succeed, the Fat Fast will be over before you know it, I promise.

An example of a quick fat-fast meal would be two ounces of cream cheese.

It's not much, but it will get you where you need to go.

The mechanics behind the Fat Fast are pretty straightforward.

You have lipolysis, which is where the body directly burns fat, and ketosis, is where the body burns ketone bodies and uses those for fuel.

These two things combined results in pretty rapid weight loss. As you might imagine, this approach is only for those who are truly "stuck".

If you're losing weight on target and your program seems to be going according to plan, then you will not have to concern yourself with the Fat Fast.

In fact, many people will go through Atkins without needing it at all.

Because this approach is high in fat, you shouldn't suffer hunger pangs while doing it.

There may well be a mental hunger as you get used to the small portions, but that doesn't mean there will to a real need to eat more than the recommended amounts (98), (99).

In my opinion, I think the Fat Fast is good approach as long as you treat it as a short term thing.

Trying to do this for long stretches (which is unnecessary anyway) will just result in you going nuts.

Trust me when I say you don't want to do this for more than about five days.

Your body will adjust as intended during this time, and then you can get back to Atkins Induction and progress forward through the remaining phases.

Up next: I am going to be talking about gallbladder issues.

One concern is whether the Atkins approach will put your gallbladder at risk. All will be revealed in chapter 33.

33 GALLBLADDER ISSUES

Have you read about how the Atkins lifestyle can mess with your gallbladder?

One of the biggest concerns that newcomers have about Atkins is that it's going to hurt their body in some way.

Some people might tell you that you're making a mistake and that the Atkins approach to eating should be avoided at all costs.

The doubters may say that it's better to go back to eating the same foods that made you feel tired and sick in the first place than it is to proceed with Atkins.

One thing that I want to do in this guide is ease your concerns on all such issues.

OK, so let's get right to it. Gallbladder issues are indeed real. The gallbladder plays a pretty strong role in the body.

It helps to break down the fat that you consume, as well as making bile (a substance essential for aiding digestion).

Fat needs to be absorbed by the body in order to be used by all the hormones.

The gallbladder is a storage organ that makes this natural process far easier than if you didn't have one. (100)

There are, at times, reasons why some people have their gallbladder removed. If you develop gallstones, then the bile gets blocked, thus preventing it from moving around to the small intestine the way it needs to.

This can be quite painful and most doctors will opt to remove the gallbladder rather than letting you live with the pain and discomfort. (101)

You might be worried that the Atkins way of eating is going to harm your gallbladder further, but this doesn't seem to be the case at all.

From what I've read, it is actually grains, sugar, and partially hydrogenated oils that tend to give the gallbladder the most trouble.

When coming off a low fat diet, then the gallbladder has to work harder because it hasn't had much work to do in terms of breaking down fats.

The best way to look at this is to think about the stress involved when going from not having a job for quite some time to having a full time position.

In effect, this is what happens with the gallbladder when switching from a low fat diet to one which is higher in fat content.

This is where trouble can really set in with Atkins if you're not cautious.

You will want to be careful and take things gradually to begin with. If you're trying to add more fat into your diet, going slowly is better than trying to cram it all in to a single meal. (102)

My point here is that there's room on the Atkins way of eating for just about anyone. Even if you don't have a gallbladder, I encourage you to start with Atkins induction.

You might have to take thing slower than someone that has a gallbladder, but even so, it is possible to accomplish your weight loss goals nonetheless.

Up next: I will be covering sleep issues that can become a problem for many low-carbers.

34 SLEEP ISSUES

There's just no other way to say it: sleep is crucial to health and wellbeing.

In fact, we just can't function properly without it.

Some people have tried, and the negative health effects are pretty devastating.

There comes a point where the mind and body just gives up and collapses into deep slumber, whether we like it or not.

I remember being so flat out busy once that when I got home it took me all my effort just to crawl into bed and flake out.

Those were not pleasant times, but they shaped me into a person who truly knows what he wants out of life.

I genuinely believe that it's time to let go of the nonstop lifestyle and allow the body to rest and rejuvenate as and when it needs to.

Getting ample sleep is a good thing, and it can make us feel and function so much better when we're up and about.

When we don't get enough sleep, the body goes into a stressed state.

When there's stress, there's cortisol, known more formally as hydrocortisone.

Cortisol is normal, and at the right dose it helps the body respond better to stress.

However, when it's at higher or more prolonged levels than normal (as with a lack of sleep), it can create a number of negative health effects, one of those being an increase in abdominal fat.

Since weight loss is what we generally want, tending to sleep is a pretty important part of our plan. (103)

A question that gets asked a lot is just how much sleep does a person really need?

The truth is that it's impossible to answer this specifically because we all require different amounts, although the general consensus is an average of eight hours quality kip per night.

Some people can leap out of bed at first light fresh and revitalized after having just four hours sleep.

Me? I'm a six hour guy, but my wife prefers to have her full eight hours.

It's just a matter of determining how much you need personally to feel great throughout the waking day, and then make that your norm. (104), (105)

It's important that you don't get your sleep piecemeal. There is a sleep cycle involved here and the more regular your sleep pattern is, the better it is for you.

You want to make sure that you're allowing the body to get the deepest sleep possible.

This is where true recovery really begins.

If you're getting nothing but shallow sleep, then your body is receiving the minimum necessary for survival.

If you were only interested in survival you wouldn't be reading this guide.

We want more than survival, a mere existence, we want quality of life, and there's absolutely nothing wrong with that. (106)

In my opinion, the quality of sleep really makes a difference.

Try not to sleep with the lights on, or in a room full of clutter, with TV and computer distractions invading your space.

You need to make sure that your bedroom is a serene area, somewhere that's clean and tidy, fresh and soothing, and most importantly, nice and dark once the lights are out.

Getting quality kip will aid in your sleep through the production of melatonin.

Melatonin is a hormone that helps to regulate sleep and wake cycles.

Also important for getting the best out of your slumber is to shut off all noises as well because even gentle background sounds can disrupt a sleep pattern.

For some of you, it might feel a little awkward at first by not sleeping with the lights dimmed or the music on, if that's how you normally drift off.

But readjusting the way you go to sleep has proved to be very beneficial for those who have broken old habits.

You might be surprised at the number of people who tell me how powerful this readjustment has been for their sleep over time. (107)

Up next: I am going to cover some mistakes that can affect men's health as it relates to the Atkins way of eating.

35 MEN'S HEALTH

The subject of men's health is actually the topic of whole volumes, and not mere chapters within books.

So if I had to pick one sub-topic that I think is timely and important as it relates to men's health, it would definitely have to be that of testosterone.

Both genders produce testosterone in the body, but it is primarily made in higher concentrations by men. In short, testosterone is the key to a man's vitality.

Testosterone is what lends to our strength, flexibility, and power.

It's behind our fertility as well.

There's quite a bit going on in terms of male hormones, so they need to be kept in check (108).

Managing testosterone is pretty important. There is such a thing as having low testosterone or low t, which is something you want to avoid.

When a man has low t, it can mess with muscle tone, mood, sex drive, and cause a general lack of energy.

If you're on the Atkins diet though, you have a natural way to really get your testosterone levels back up. (109)

Not only do you have the right diet on your side, you also have exercise to help.

A study done by the famous low carb researcher Dr. Jeff Volek, indicates that there is a connection between higher levels of testosterone and regular exercise.

The study was published in the Journal of Applied Physiology, back in January 1997. It's an older study, but it's still interesting nonetheless.

We often think that we need to do a whole bunch of stuff in order to improve our health, but in truth, for most of us, it's as simple as eating well and exercising regularly. (110)

It's important to point out here that many physical and emotional symptoms are shared by numerous health conditions.

If you're not feeling the way you should do, there's a good chance your diet could be upsetting the balance.

You need to ask yourself whether you're really reaching for variety, or just going with a lot of low carb convenience food that isn't serving your best interests.

Whether you've started on Atkins, or about to begin your journey, if you don't feel as well as you should do, then it goes without saying that you should consult your doctor without delay.

Self-diagnosis (aside from the obvious), and particularly self-treatment, can be a dangerous thing and should never be messed with.

Remember: eat well and exercise regularly.

These are two mistakes I made on my journey as I looked for shortcuts, and I just don't want them to happen to you too.

Up next: In the next chapter I will be covering a few health related issues for the ladies.

36 WOMEN'S HEALTH

Just as testosterone is one of the primary hormones we focus on in men, it's estrogen that we concentrate on in women.

When estrogen levels are unusually high, heart issues, obesity, and high blood pressure are often up there as well.

When testosterone levels are too high in women, then hair growth can get out of control resulting in male pattern baldness and unwelcome growth on the upper lip and chin. (111)

The key to life is balance, and I find that the Atkins Nutritional Approach does a good job of attaining balance in women.

My wife struggled with moodiness and fatigue for a long time.

When I announced I would be starting the Atkins diet, and pointed out how it can help repair and maintain both physical and emotional health, she was intrigued.

She also had a little stubborn weight that she wanted to lose, so we decided to try the Atkins approach together.

I wasn't prepared for the way the diet affected her mood.

Without any exaggeration, her irritability faded away as she entered ketosis, and we're both so grateful for that!

I'm finding more and more issues being treated well on a low carb diet too.

For example, the Atkins Nutritional Approach has shown to have a positive effect on polycystic ovarian syndrome (PCOS); one of the top hormonal issues in women today.

A study published in December 2005 in the Nutrition & Metabolism Journal connected PCOS with obesity as well as insulin resistance; two things that make it really hard for women to lose weight (112).

The study found that a ketogenic diet (which is very much like the Atkins Induction phase) actually led to improvements in the ability to lose weight, and hormonal profiles too.

Could you be out of balance right now?

If you think there's a possibility then you need to get to your doctor's office as soon as possible.

If you suspect that you have PCOS, a low carb diet approach is definitely helpful, but do speak with a medical professional first.

A doctor may also want to prescribe certain medications to help with the overall battle, and it's important to follow whatever advice is given.

Conventional medication coupled with the Atkins diet has shown to be a great way to manage the symptoms of PCOS, but like I say, do not make any lifestyle changes without first consulting your doctor.

Up next: I will be talking about pregnancy and the Atkins diet. Bringing new life into the world is a pretty special thing, and something we need to look at.

37 PREGNANCY

As a researcher, pregnancy is one of my favorite topics.

Since we've been around for thousands upon thousands of years, it's no surprise that there has been a lot of research conducted around this prenatal period.

If you're on a low carb diet like Atkins, then you will want to read some of the strong science that backs up why the low carb diet is a good choice.

If you are worried about gestational diabetes, for example, let me put your mind at ease. When women get pregnant, the body becomes a little bit insulin resistant.

This is actually nature's way of protecting the unborn child.

If you weren't at least a little insulin resistant during pregnancy, your body would seize nutrients faster than the baby, bringing in the risk of defects through lack of nutrition.

Instead, nature decided to make sure that the unborn gets nourished as it develops, even at the cost of the mother's nutritional needs.

A pregnant woman can become half-starved, almost literally, yet the baby remains unharmed. This is nature's way of ensuring the survival of the next generation. (113)

I also came across a study published in the American Journal of Physiology. It indicates that a baby "remembers" obesity through the mother. It sounds weird, but it's going into a part of science called epigenetics.

If this is a little over your head don't worry, I'll attempt to explain it in layman's terms.

It took me a while to fully understand what's going on, but it clicked in the end.

The study confirms that when an expectant mother is obese, inflammation is also present within the body, and the growing baby inside the pregnant woman picks up on this obesity.

The result of this is that there's a strong likelihood that the child will also become obese later on in life.

OK, so this means that being on a low carb diet, we're teaching a much more even blood sugar pattern than the hectic need to feed every few hours.

That's the beauty of running on fat because you don't have to manage your days making sure you're always within close proximity to food in the same chaotic way.

Naturally, you will still need to fuel your body as a pregnant woman.

Getting plenty of healthy fat is absolutely essential for the baby's growing brain and body. You also want to make sure that you're getting in some protein too.

Now, I know that morning sickness is an issue in the first trimester of pregnancy, but try not to worry about it. Eat what you're able to and resolve to get back to Atkins as soon as you can.

I don't recommend "Induction" per se, but if you do have to go with the Phase One style of eating, then that's perfectly fine. (114)

Up next: I want to talk about depression issues connected to low carb living as it relates to Atkins specifically.

38 DEPRESSION ISSUES

A popular commercial for a depression drug has a tagline that stuck in my mind.

It goes: "Depression Hurts".

We often refer to depression as being in the blues, but in truth it can be a lot more serious than just feeling down in the dumps.

Individuals experience depression with varying intensity and there is no "standard" for the condition.

Some people feel it in a way that doesn't really hit them too hard or for too long, that is, with a little effort they can shrug it off and keep on functioning.

But clinical depression often goes way beyond this.

It can feel next to impossible to lift the mood, even to fake it.

It can become so bad in some people, that they may not even have the energy to try. (115)

One treatment that seems helpful with depression is cod liver oil.

If you're going to try this, then I recommend buying only the highest quality oil you can find.

This is definitely not a time where you want to skimp by purchasing substandard oils.

Remember, this is going into your body, so it definitely matters what type of oil you choose.

I like fermented cod liver oil as it really delivers the benefits you're looking for.

Something as prevalent as depression needs to be taken as seriously as possible. (116)

If you have already been diagnosed and prescribed anti-depressants, it's important that you don't suddenly stop taking them just because you've gone low carb with the Atkins Nutritional Approach.

Coming off medication suddenly can be dangerous in some cases, and that just wouldn't make sense at all.

A lot of depression-related medications have serious side effects if the patient stops taking them overnight, so it's crucial that you speak with your doctor first if you would like to wean off or cut back on your tablets. (117)

Up next: Here we will go into one of our final lessons and look at –"net carbohydrates"

39 NET CARBS

If you're just starting out then you have probably realized that one of the hardest mistakes to avoid is ascertaining the difference between "net carbs" and "total carbs."

In simple terms, a net carbohydrate is the result after taking the fiber out of the carbohydrate listing on the labels of your food. (118)

Let's use an avocado as an example.

If you take an avocado and start reading down the nutritional facts, you might become a little concerned when you see 13 grams of carbs.

That can be quite a bit if you're on Atkins Induction.

However, all is not as it seems.

When net carbs are calculated, there is only a carb count of 3g for a cup of cubed avocado.

That should definitely put you at ease and make you more enthusiastic about this way of eating. (119)

Believe me when I say I know just how daunting this can seem as a newcomer.

When I first began this way of eating, I became increasingly worried that there wasn't going to be much at all that I could actually eat.

I started going round in circles at the grocery store because I was concerned that those carbs were just going to sneak up on me in most foods.

If you focus on those things that have some fiber in them, you might be surprised at how low carb some of these items are.

On the later phases of Atkins, you can add beans back into your diet because by now you would have tested what's going to work for your body and what isn't.

Does this mean you have to rush the process?

No, not at all!

There are some people who actually count total carbs over net carbs, but this is not something Dr. Atkins talks about too much in "Dr. Atkins New Diet Revolution" or any of his later books. It's going to be up to you.

I recommend sticking with net carbs because that's "strict" Atkins.

On the other hand, if you feel that your weight loss isn't moving as well as you hoped, then you can limit yourself based on the total carbs count.

What I've found helps to keep me in check when it comes to carbs, is to get in as much fat as I can stand.

A higher consumption of fat definitely makes me feel less hungry, and that means that I'm not raiding the fridge at odd hours of the day and night curbing hunger pangs.

Just know that when you get things right, there's plenty of great benefits waiting for you within the world of Atkins!

Next up: Chapter 40, our final chapter. This is where I tie everything together and get you started on the best path possible!

40 ACTION STEPS FOR YOUR NEW ATKINS LIFE

OK, so you have reached the last chapter, so well done for sticking with it.

This series is very near and dear to my heart, and I want you to know how much I truly care about the health and wellbeing of my readers.

For me, that's exactly why I write and continue talking about these topics.

Please know that if there's anything I can do for you, any question I can answer, feel free to send it my way.

Digging into the science is great, but more and more people are asking me how to tie all these things together. In short, they feel lost, overwhelmed, and hesitant

The first basic principle is to start in your kitchen and clear away all those food items that don't support your diet.

Removing temptation, especially in the early days, is fundamental to starting on the right footing.

I write about the "big kitchen clean out" a lot, simply because I think it's absolutely critical.

If you have an unhealthy attachment to food, then there is little chance you will be able to just skip over the wrong foods while reaching out for the right items.

There is nothing wrong with admitting that you have a problem with food.

Denial is a major hurdle for a lot of people wanting to lose weight and live a healthier, happier lifestyle.

But it is only when we can see things for what they really are that we have a real fighting chance to correct them. Some people skip over their relationship with food entirely, but I think that's silly.

It's much better to admit to any problems with food, and then hold the head up high and march forwards.

To every problem there is a solution, but the solution can only be sought when the problem is identified.

The Atkins Nutritional Approach will give you the tools you need to achieve your goals.

Out of all the low carb diets around today, I truly feel that this is the one which really gives people the best and most sustainable outcome.

Atkins may start off a little harsh, but it evens out to the point where you get to determine just how many carbs you can handle, and how many you're going to have to restrict.

It lets you identify what food intolerances you have and helps you to really become familiar with your own body.

Some people might find that they have to avoid dairy, and for others it may be wheat.

Either way, it will be you who discovers those things that you need to cut down on or completely remove from your diet.

It's all good here, and providing you follow the instructions methodically, you will find that there's a seat at the Atkins table for you too.

There is something special about being able to eat well, enjoy food, and still see weight loss.

But it's not just about weight loss, as you have learned throughout in this guide.

As well as maintaining a healthy weight, I want you to sleep better, live better, and function better from the inside out.

I want you to overcome depression, vastly reduce the risk of heart health issues, and everything else that's associated with an unhealthy lifestyle. Isn't that what we all want?

Well now you can have it.

If you can, find yourself a support group filled with like-minded people.

They will help you to stay on track and keep focused when others are telling you what a terrible diet you're on.

And if you have time, really check out some of the studies referenced in the footnotes.

These studies make for a really interesting read.

Furthermore, they will give you a bit of "ammo" to use in any discussions you might have with co-workers, friends, and family members who negatively debate the Atkins approach without having the facts.

From here on in the world is your oyster! Go shopping and get stocked up on food items that pertain to whichever Atkins phase you are on.

I'm in your corner here, and wish you all the very best as you progress forwards on your journey to a better way of living.

REFERENCES

1. National Center for Health Statistics. (2004). Health, United States, 2004 with chartbook on trends in the health of Americans. Hyattsville, MD: Author.
2. http://www.ncbi.nlm.nih.gov/pmc/articles/PMC1126011/
3. http://www.webmd.com/diet/features/give-your-pantry-a-healthy-makeover
4. http://lowcarbdiets.about.com/od/atkinsdiet/p/atkins1.htm
5. http://lowcarbdiets.about.com/od/whattoeat/a/packagedfood.htm
6. http://www.nytimes.com/2011/04/17/magazine/mag-17Sugar-t.html?pagewanted=all&_r=0
7. http://lowcarbdiets.about.com/od/atkinsdiet/a/inductionoption.htm
8. http://lowcarbdiets.about.com/od/atkinsdiet/p/atkins1.htm
9. http://www.ketogenic-diet-resource.com/ketoacidosis.html
10. http://www.marksdailyapple.com/low-carb-flu/
11. http://www.rpi.edu/dept/bcbp/molbiochem/MBWeb/mb1/part2/gluconeo
12. http://www.ext.colostate.edu/pubs/foodnut/09315.html
13. http://wholehealthsource.blogspot.com/2009/12/butyric-acid-ancient-controller-of.html
14. http://www.gnolls.org/3374/there-is-no-such-thing-as-a-calorie-to-your-body/
15. http://garytaubes.com/2011/09/catching-up-on-lost-time-ancestral-health-symposium-food-reward-palatability-insulin-signaling-carbohydrates-kettles-pots-other-odds-ends-part-i/
16. http://www.mayoclinic.com/health/atkins-diet/my00648
17. http://scoobysworkshop.com/how-to-weigh-yourself-accurately/
18. http://www.healthdiscovery.net/articles/scale_lies.htm
19. http://www.huffingtonpost.com/2013/07/25/myths-facts-weight-loss_n_3611969.html
20. http://www.fitday.com/fitness-articles/nutrition/fats/heart-health-does-saturated-fat-clog-arteries.html
21. http://www.askdrsears.com/topics/family-nutrition/facts-about-fats/why-you-need-fats
22. http://ajcn.nutrition.org/content/early/2010/08/04/ajcn.2009.29146.abstract
23. http://www.huffingtonpost.com/dr-mark-hyman/why-cholesterol-may-not-b_b_290687.html
24. http://rejuvandwellbeing.com/the-atkins-diet
25. http://diabetes.niddk.nih.gov/dm/pubs/insulinresistance/
26. http://www.nhlbi.nih.gov/health/health-topics/topics/ms/
27. http://lowcarbconfidential.com/2007/07/04/atkins-induction-observations-on-my-first-few-days/

28. http://www.atkins.com/Science/Articles---Library/Atkins-Lifestyle-(1)/Reach-Your-Goal-by-Climbing-the-Carb-Ladder.aspx
29. http://ajpendo.physiology.org/content/292/6/E1724.full
30. http://lowcarbdiets.about.com/od/atkinsdiet/p/atkins2.htm
31. http://www.atkins.com/Program/Phase-2.aspx
32. http://www.atkins.com/Program/Phase-2/Trouble-Shooting-in-OWL.aspx
33. http://lowcarbdiets.about.com/od/atkinsdiet/p/atkins3.htm
34. http://www.cnpp.usda.gov/dgas2010-dgacreport.htm
35. http://www.cdc.gov/nccdphp/dnpa/nutrition/pdf/portion_size_research.pdf
36. http://www.lowcarb.ca/tips/tips008.html
37. http://www.atkins.com/Program/Phase-4.aspx
38. http://onlinelibrary.wiley.com/doi/10.1111/j.1467-789X.2005.00170.x/abstract?deniedAccessCustomisedMessage=&userIsAuthenticated=false
39. http://www.mayoclinic.com/health/anaphylaxis/DS00009
40. http://www.mayoclinic.com/health/food-allergy/AN01109
41. http://drhyman.com/blog/2010/04/20/are-your-food-allergies-making-you-fat/
42. http://www.gnolls.org/3224/dietary-protein-101-what-is-protein-and-why-do-we-need-to-eat-it-every-day/
43. http://www.atkins.com/Program/Overview/How-and-Why-Atkins-Work/Atkins-Is-Not-a-High-Protein-Diet.aspx
44. http://lowcarb4u.blogspot.com/2009/07/how-can-eating-excess-protein-raise.html
45. http://kidney.niddk.nih.gov/kudiseases/pubs/yourkidneys/
46. http://cjasn.asnjournals.org/content/early/2012/05/30/CJN.11741111.abstract
47. http://articles.mercola.com/sites/articles/archive/2010/04/20/sugar-dangers.aspx
48. http://www.lowcarb.ca/tips/tips006.html
49. http://www.thestar.com/life/health_wellness/2013/07/30/dont_drink_your_calories_mayo_clinic.html
50. http://www.foodandhealing.com/articles/article-wholefoods.htm
51. http://wellnessmama.com/5356/cravings-fix-your-leptin/
52. http://www.ncbi.nlm.nih.gov/pmc/articles/PMC33319/
53. http://articles.mercola.com/sites/articles/archive/2012/10/29/leptin-resistance.aspx
54. http://www.ncbi.nlm.nih.gov/pubmed/23700076
55. http://www.webmd.com/diet/features/the-facts-on-leptin-faq
56. http://ajcn.nutrition.org/content/early/2013/06/26/ajcn.113.064113.abstract
57. http://www.ncbi.nlm.nih.gov/books/NBK53550/
58. http://www.ncbi.nlm.nih.gov/pubmed/7631905
59. http://www.ncbi.nlm.nih.gov/pubmed/1568575
60. http://www.ncbi.nlm.nih.gov/pubmed/2375420
61. http://lowcarbdiets.about.com/od/lowcarb101/ss/How-To-Cut-Carbs-Web-Version-of-Ecourse_12.htm
62. http://link.springer.com/article/10.1007%2FBF02533732
63. http://www.mayoclinic.com/health/trans-fat/CL00032
64. http://www.mayoclinic.com/health/hypothyroidism/DS00353
65. http://www.stopthethyroidmadness.com/iodine12345/
66. http://www.mayoclinic.com/health/hyperthyroidism/DS00344
67. http://www.livestrong.com/article/412216-will-bananas-raise-blood-sugar/
68. http://healthyfitmom.com/potassium-rich-low-carb-foods/
69. http://www.emedicinehealth.com/low_potassium/article_em.htm
70. http://www.fitday.com/fitness-articles/nutrition/vitamins-minerals/potassium-why-its-essential-for-your-body.html
71. http://www.healthyandorganic.com/magnesium.html
72. Rubin H. Central role for magnesium in coordinate control of metabolism and growth in animal cells. Proceedings of the National Academy of Sciences of the USA. 1975 Sep;72(9):3551-5.
73. http://www.medscape.com/viewarticle/423568
74. http://www.fitday.com/fitness-articles/nutrition/vitamins-minerals/vitamin-d-why-its-important.html#b

75. http://www.niams.nih.gov/Health_Info/Bone/Bone_Health/Nutrition/
76. http://www.mayoclinic.com/health/vitamin-d/NS_patient-vitamind
77. http://ods.od.nih.gov/factsheets/Calcium-QuickFacts/
78. http://www.medicalnewstoday.com/articles/248958.php
79. http://ajcn.nutrition.org/content/37/6/924.short
80. http://holdthetoast.com/node/28
81. http://www.cabdirect.org/abstracts/19801408535.html;jsessionid=0E8FBE429F068E838DD67E1863DEAA6C
82. http://jama.jamanetwork.com/article.aspx?articleid=414802
83. http://www.nlm.nih.gov/medlineplus/ency/article/002422.htm
84. http://www.seasalthealth.com/2012/04/11/health-benefits-of-sea-salt/
85. http://www.scientificamerican.com/article.cfm?id=its-time-to-end-the-war-on-salt
86. http://lowcarbdiets.about.com/b/2013/05/26/should-we-worry-about-salt.htm
87. http://eurheartj.oxfordjournals.org/content/34/14/1034.abstract/reply#ehj_el_1743
88. http://www.mayoclinic.com/health/fiber/NU00033
89. http://jama.jamanetwork.com/article.aspx?articleid=190211
90. http://ajcn.nutrition.org/content/25/9/926.short
91. http://www.mayoclinic.com/health/caffeine/NU00600
92. http://livinlavidalocarb.blogspot.com/2007/08/does-caffeine-impact-ketosis-on-low.html
93. http://well.blogs.nytimes.com/2011/12/14/how-coffee-can-galvanize-your-workout/?_r=0
94. http://lowcarbdiets.about.com/od/whattoeat/a/alcbev.htm
95. http://www2.potsdam.edu/hansondj/HealthIssues/1110385823.html
96. http://www.psychologytoday.com/blog/addiction-in-society/201011/science-is-what-society-says-it-is-alcohols-poison
97. http://www.carbsmart.com/fatfast.html
98. http://www.ncbi.nlm.nih.gov/pmc/articles/PMC3031774/
99. http://www.plosbiology.org/article/info%3Adoi%2F10.1371%2Fjournal.pbio.1001485
100. http://www.zocdoc.com/answers/9890/what-does-the-gall-bladder-do
101. http://www.webmd.com/digestive-disorders/tc/gallstones-topic-overview
102. http://www.atkins.com/Science/Articles---Library/General-Health-Issues/Dealing-with-Gallbladder-Disorders.aspx
103. http://www.naturalmedicinejournal.com/article_content.asp?article=93
104. http://www.sleepfoundation.org/article/how-sleep-works/how-much-sleep-do-we-really-need
105. http://www.mayoclinic.com/health/sleep/HQ01387
106. http://www.sleepforall.com/sleep-cycle.htm
107. http://healthland.time.com/2013/02/08/sleeping-it-off-how-alcohol-affects-sleep-quality/
108. http://www.news-medical.net/health/Testosterone-Physiological-Effects.aspx
109. http://www.nlm.nih.gov/medlineplus/tutorials/lowtestosterone/ur189103.pdf
110. http://jap.physiology.org/content/82/1/49.full
111. http://women.webmd.com/guide/normal-testosterone-and-estrogen-levels-in-women?page=2
112. http://www.ncbi.nlm.nih.gov/pmc/articles/PMC1334192/
113. http://www.ncbi.nlm.nih.gov/pubmed/378620
114. http://ajpregu.physiology.org/content/early/2010/07/14/ajpregu.00310.2010
115. http://www.mayoclinic.com/health/clinical-depression/AN01057
116. http://www.ncbi.nlm.nih.gov/pubmed/17184843
117. http://www.mypassion4health.com/articles/amino_acid_therapy.html
118. http://lowcarbdiets.about.com/od/products/a/netcarbs.htm
119. http://nutritiondata.self.com/facts/fruits-and-fruit-juices/1843/2

ABOUT THE AUTHOR

Mirsad writes all of his books in a unique style, constantly drawing connections between his past experiences and his reader's goals. This unique approach means that you can avoid undergoing the same injuries, frustrations, and setbacks that he himself has endured over the years. He can't produce the results for you, but what he can do is promise that you WILL reach your goals - guaranteed – providing you follow his tips and advice exactly as he outlines them in his books.

Made in the USA
Lexington, KY
29 September 2014